AIS90

The Abbreviated Injury Scale 1990 Revision

Update 98
日本語対訳版

監訳
日本外傷学会
財団法人 日本自動車研究所

翻訳
日本外傷学会 Trauma registry 検討委員会

へるす出版

Copyright © 1998 the Association for the Advancement of Automotive Medicine
Japanese translation rights arranged with the Association for the Advancement of Automotive Medicine through Japan Automobile Research Institute

AIS90 Update98 日本語対訳版出版にあたって

　本書は，米国自動車医学振興協会（Association for the Advancement of Automotive Medicine；AAAM）が刊行している最新版の Abbreviated Injury Scale（AIS），1990 Revised Version：Update 98の日本語対訳版です。AIS は，1971年米国において，自動車交通事故のさいに人体に生じた損傷をスケール化するために開発されたものです。AIS は医学あるいは自動車工学の関係者のみならず，自動車交通事故の調査研究や自動車の安全性向上にかかわる人々にきわめて有益であり，最近では主要国において翻訳され広く活用され始めています。AIS の起源とその歴史的変遷は本書の序文を読んでいただくこととして，日本における AIS 邦訳の歴史は次のような経過をたどっています。

　日本における AIS の翻訳は1980年版の AIS80が最初でした。この翻訳は自動車交通事故における人体の被害軽減にかかわるデータをより的確に把握し，より一層の自動車安全性の向上を目指すことを目的として，1983年に日本交通科学協議会に所属する医学ならびに工学の専門家の協力を得て行われました。しかしながら，この当時においては，AIS の活用は非常に限定されていました。そのため，AIS の翻訳も，広く刊行物として公表することまでは考えず，関係者内部における活用資料とする条件で AAAM から翻訳許諾を得ました。さらに，1990年には AIS の改訂版が発行されました。その当時，旧運輸省は自動車安全性のさらなる向上のための事故例調査解析の拡大と同時に，国際的な事故データの比較やこれをもとにした国際基準のハーモナイゼイションなどを求めていました。このような状況をふまえて，この事故例調査の推進には，国際的な標準化を図るための人体傷害度スケールが必要となりました。旧運輸省の事故例調査の推進母体であった（財）日本自動車研究所と筑波大学法医学教室が中心となり，日本交通科学協議会の成果を引き継いで，AAAM から翻訳許諾を得て AIS90の翻訳を行いました。（財）日本自動車研究所はこの AIS90を活用して，実際の自動車交通外傷の損傷形態から外傷重症度としての Injury Severity Score（ISS）などを計算し，自動車事故における人体の損傷状況の分析などを行っていました。しかし，まだ医学面からの本格的な活用は普及しておらず，車両の破損程度とその事故によって被った人体の損傷程度との関係がどのように定量化できるかなど工学的な面からの活用が主体となっていました。

　最近の IT 技術を駆使した自動車の安全構造・装備などの開発技術の高度化による安全対策効果とその評価には，その対策技術と人体損傷との関連について一貫して解析できる情報システムの構築が求められています。しかし，従来のマクロ統計事故データでは，これらの情報が死亡，重症，軽症という非常に大括りで分析されているのみで，交通事故における自動車の安全対策には不十分でした。人体の損傷メカニズムが推測可能な情報として損傷の向き・大きさ・内容などがわかる詳細な損傷データの AIS コーディングが是非，必要となってきております。

　このような機会に，日本外傷学会との連携により，最新版の『AIS90 Update98』の翻訳を出版できることとなりました。本書の出版により，全国的な Trauma registry データベースの構築できる基礎が確立されることは，「自動車交通事故の研究が安全の基盤」であるとして取り組んでいる工学者にとってはまさに時期を得た活動といえ，今後の自動車の安全性の飛躍的な向上に結びつくものと確信しております。

財団法人 日本自動車研究所
AIS 翻訳チーム
世話人　小野　古志郎

訳者序文

　1974年Bakerらにより提唱されたInjury Severity Score (ISS) は，解剖学的な外傷重症度を決定するための世界的な標準となっています。ISSの計算は米国自動車医学振興協会（Association for the Advancement of Automotive Medicine；AAAM）が刊行しているAbbreviated Injury Scale (AIS) に基づいた重症度スコアによっています。交通事故調査チームのための損傷スケール化を目的に1971年に発表されたAISは，これまで数回の改訂を経た結果，交通事故に限らず，穿通性外傷を含むすべての損傷形態を対象とした重症度スケールへと発展してきました。最新版の『AIS90 Update98』（本書）ではコード体系は構造的に統合，洗練され，コード選択にさいしての注意書きも充実しています。また，ISS算出の基本的ルールも記載されています。

　さて，日本外傷学会では，重症外傷患者治療の標準的なプロセスとアウトカムを収集したデータバンクを構築し，外傷治療の質の向上をはかる目的で，全国的なTrauma registry（外傷患者登録）の導入を目指しています。これまでわが国では日常臨床上，頻度の高い損傷については，AISスコアだけを知る目的で，部位別・臓器別の簡便なAISスコア表を用いていたと思われます。しかし，Trauma registryではすべての損傷について，本書に基づいてコードを適切に選択することと，ISS算出のルールを知っておくことが必要です。

　『AIS90 Update98』は，すでに（財）日本自動車研究所により翻訳権が取得され，翻訳作業が行われていましたが，草稿を拝見したところ，臨床医が使用するには医学的表現や訳語が不十分であると思われました。このため，Trauma registry検討委員会は外傷の専門家の立場から，解説文を含めすべての損傷形態の訳語の見直しと訂正作業を数カ月以上にわたって行いました。日米の用語の対応は，基本的に日本外傷学会用語委員会編集による『外傷用語集』との整合性をもたせるように心掛け，いくつかの頻出する用語の対訳については別掲の表にまとめました。また，損傷形態の英語表記を残し対訳にすることで，「手引書（dictionary）」の使用者が原文も参考にして，より正確に損傷名とそのコードを選択できるようにしました。損傷形態の一部に米国外傷外科学会のOrgan Injury Scale (OIS) が併記されていますが，詳細はインターネットURL：http://www.aast.org/injury/injury.htmlを参照してください。

　本書が外傷患者を診療する多くの医師と自動車事故研究者らに利用され，わが国におけるTrauma registryの成功と外傷学の発展，さらに自動車安全性の向上と外傷予防に寄与することを願っています。

平成15年9月

日本外傷学会 Trauma registry 検討委員会
委員長　小関　一英

目　　次

1998 Update について …………………………………………………………………………… 7

はじめに
 1．AIS の起源 ……………………………………………………………………………… 9
 2．AIS の目的と概念 ……………………………………………………………………… 9
 3．多発外傷の評価 ………………………………………………………………………… 10
 4．ICD と AIS の互換性 ………………………………………………………………… 10

AIS90における改良点
 1．コード選択のガイドライン …………………………………………………………… 11
 2．穿通性損傷 ……………………………………………………………………………… 11
 3．小児外傷 ………………………………………………………………………………… 11
 4．損傷リストの拡張 ……………………………………………………………………… 12
 5．損傷コードの見方 ……………………………………………………………………… 12
 6．体表損傷 ………………………………………………………………………………… 12
 7．脳損傷 …………………………………………………………………………………… 12
 8．用語の修正と変更 ……………………………………………………………………… 13

まとめ ………………………………………………………………………………………………… 14

References ……………………………………………………………………………………………… 15

手引書の使い方
 1．様式 ……………………………………………………………………………………… 17
 2．コード選択のルール …………………………………………………………………… 17
 3．ISS（Injury Severity Score）の計算 ………………………………………………… 21
   A．一般的なルール …………………………………………………………………… 21
   B．皮膚損傷のコード選択 …………………………………………………………… 22

手引書
 頭　部 ……………………………………………………………………………………… 23
 顔　面 ……………………………………………………………………………………… 33
 頸　部 ……………………………………………………………………………………… 36
 胸　部 ……………………………………………………………………………………… 39
 腹部および骨盤内臓器 …………………………………………………………………… 46
 脊　椎
  頸　椎 …………………………………………………………………………………… 55
  胸　椎 …………………………………………………………………………………… 58
  腰　椎 …………………………………………………………………………………… 60
 上　肢 ……………………………………………………………………………………… 62
 下　肢 ……………………………………………………………………………………… 67
 体表，熱傷，他の外傷
  体表－皮膚および皮下組織 …………………………………………………………… 73
  熱　傷 …………………………………………………………………………………… 74
  他の外傷 ………………………………………………………………………………… 76

 索　引 ……………………………………………………………………………………… 77

頻出用語対応表（アルファベット順）

Abrasion	擦過傷
Avulsion	剥離（皮膚），断裂（皮膚以外）
Comminuted	粉砕
Contusion	挫傷
Crush	挫滅
Destruction	高度損傷
Displaced	転位
Disruption	破壊，離断
Extensive	広範囲
Intimal tear	内膜剥離
Laceration	裂創（皮膚），裂傷・裂創（皮膚以外）
Large	多量
Major	大
Massive	大量
Massive destruction	広範囲損傷
Minor	小
Open	開放
Perforation	穿孔
Puncture	穿刺
Small	少量
Transection	離断，断裂

●訳　者

〔日本外傷学会 Trauma registry 検討委員会〕

小関　一英（委員長）：川口市立医療センター救命救急センター長
齋藤　大蔵：防衛医科大学校救急部講師
坂本　哲也：帝京大学救命救急センター教授
東平日出夫：大阪府立泉州救命救急センター
藤田　　尚：帝京大学救命救急センター
益子　邦洋：日本医科大学付属千葉北総病院救命救急センター長
森村　尚登：帝京大学救命救急センター講師
横田順一朗：大阪府立泉州救命救急センター所長

〔財団法人日本自動車研究所 AIS 翻訳チーム〕

小野古志郎（世話人）：財団法人日本自動車研究所主席研究員
岩楯　公晴：元筑波大学社会医学系法医学（現東京医科歯科大学講師）
大橋　教良：筑波メディカルセンター病院副院長
大橋　秀幸：財団法人日本自動車研究所主任研究員（財団法人交通事故総合分析センター出向つくば交通事
　　　　　　故調査事務所所長代理）
河野　元嗣：筑波メディカルセンター病院救急総合診療部部長
丹野　高三：元筑波大学社会医学系法医学（現弘前大学医学部法医学助手）
三澤　章吾：前筑波大学社会医学系法医学教授（現東京都監察医務院院長）

1998 Update について

1998年に行われた AIS90 の改訂では，次のような基本的な目標を達成した。

　第一に，手引書（dictionary）全体にわたって広範囲に及ぶコード選択のルールと取り扱い方を提示した。このため前の版に比べて容易にコード選択を行うことができるようになった。AIS90にもコード選択のためのガイドラインが含まれていたが，この98年改訂版ではより一層充実したものとなった。
　第二に，とくに体表損傷に対する ISS 計算のルールを明確にした。
　第三に，米国外傷外科学会（American Association for the Surgery of Trauma：AAST）が開発した臓器損傷スケール（Organ Injury Scale：OIS）を導入したことである。このスケールは AIS90 に記述されている損傷形態の表現によく合致している。本来，OIS は胸部および腹部の損傷に合致すると考えられていた。OIS を導入することにより，臨床研究に AIS を広く適用できるようになると期待される。

　損傷スケーリング委員会（Committee on Injury Scaling）は，AIS の利用にあたり基本原則が確実に守られているかに注目している。AIS の利用者は，技術的背景がそれぞれ異なること，重症度についてのデータにさまざまなニーズがあること，また，外傷情報を入手する方法にも多様性があることを考慮して，標準化したコード選択ルールを採用している。このように利用者の意図はさまざまであっても，この AIS98年改訂版に統合されたルールを忠実に適用すれば，外傷データを適切なレベルで比較することが可能になる。このコード選択ルールから逸脱すれば，外傷重症度の研究結果は疑わしいものになるだろう。

ACKNOWLEDGEMENTS

The AIS has gained global recognition over the years due to the efforts of many individuals. Those who directly contributed to the several revisions are listed here followed by those who provided valuable input to the 1998 update.

Members of the Committee on Injury Scaling (1973 through 1990*):
* Thomas A. Gennarelli, M.D., Professor of Neurosurgery, University of Pennsylvania (Chairman)
* Elaine Petrucelli, Executive Director, Association for the Advancement of Automotive Medicine
* Susan P. Baker, M.P.H., Professor of Health Policy and Management, Johns Hopkins University
  Robert W. Bryant, Accident Investigation, General Motors Research Laboratories, Warren ,MI
* Howard R, Champion, M.D., Chief of Trauma Services, Washington Hospital Center
* Stephen A. Deane, M.D., Senior Lecturer in Surgery, Sydney University, Australia
* Harold A. Fenner, M.D., Orthopedic Surgeon, Hobbs, NM
  Robert N. Green, M.D., LLB, Coroner, Province of Ontario, Canada (retired)
  Michael Henderson, M.D., Australian Doctors' Fund, Sydney, Australia
  A.C. Hering, M.D., Secretary, Committee on Trauma, American College of Surgeons, Chicago, IL (retired)
* Donald F. Huelke, Ph,D., Professor of Anatomy and Cell Biology, University of Michigan
* Ellen J. MacKenzie, Ph.D., Associate Professor of Health Policy and Management, Johns Hopkins University
  Joseph C. Marsh, Research Engineer, Ford Motor Co., Dearborn, MI
* Gerri M. McGinnis, M.S.N., Associate Director, Head Injury Center, University of Pennsylvania
  Kermit Morgan, Staff Engineer, American Motors, Detroit, MI (retired)
* John A. Morris, Jr., M.D., Assistant Professor of Surgery, Vanderbilt University
  W.D. Nelson, General Motors Technical Center, Warren, MI (retired)
  J. Thomas Noga, NASS Program, National Highway Traffic Safety Administration, U.S. Dept. of Transportation
* John E. Pless, M.D., Professor of Pathology, Indiana University
  W.J. Ruby, Staff Engineer, Ford Motor Co., Dearborn, MI (retired)
  G. Anthony Ryan, M.D., Road Accident Research Unit, University of Adelaide
* John D. States, M.D., Professor Emeritus of Orthopedics, University of Rochester
* Joseph J. Tepas, III, M.D., Associate Professor of Pediatric Surgery, University of Florida
* Donald D. Trunkey, M.D., Professor of Surgery, Oregon Health Sciences University
* David C. Viano, Ph.D., Biomedical Science Department, General Motors Research Laboratories
* David W. Yates, M.D., Senior Lecturer, Accident & Emergency Medicine, Manchester UK

American College of Surgeons' Advisors:
William F. Blaisdell, M.D., Professor of Surgery, University of California, Davis
Charles F. Frey, M.D., Professor of Surgery, University of California, San Francisco
Frank R. Lewis, M.D., Professor of Surgery, University of California, San Francisco

American Association for the Surgery of Trauma Advisor:
Eugene Moore, M.D, Professor of Surgery, University of Colorado, Denver

Pediatric Surgical Panel Advisors:
J. Alex Haller, M.D., Professor of Pediatric Surgery, Johns Hopkins University
Burton H. Harris, M.D., Professor of Pediatric Surgery, New England Medical Center, Boston
Michael E. Matlack, M.D., Professor of Pediatric Surgery, University of Utah
Max L. Ramenofsky, M.D., Professor of Pediatric Surgery, University of Pittsburgh
David E. Wesson, M.D., Associate Professor of Pediatric Surgery, Toronto Sick Childrens Hospital
Bonnie L. Beaver, M.D., Assistant Professor of Surgery, University of Maryland Hospital, Baltimore

Ad Hoc Advisors:
Leonard M. Parver, M.D., Associate Professor of Ophthalmology, Georgetown University
Richard C. Schultz, M.D., Professor of Plastic and Reconstructive Surgery, University of Illinois

Injury Scaling Review Panel for 98 Update:
Thomas A. Gennarelli, M.D., Professor of Neurosurgery, Allegheny University
Jeffrey S. Augenstein, M.D., Professor of Surgery, University of Miami
Howard Champion, M.D., Director of Research, Program and Trauma, University of Maryland
Brad Cushing, M.D., Director, Trauma & Surgical Critical Care, Maine Medical Center
Thomas Esposito, M.D., Assistant Director, Burn and Shock Trauma Institute, Loyola University
Peter L. Lane, M.D., Director of Clinical Research, Albert Einstein Medical Center
Ellen MacKenzie, Ph.D., Professor of Health Policy and Management, Johns Hopkins University
Gerri McGinnis, Ph.D., Department of Neurosurgery, Allegheny University
Elaine Petrucelli, Executive Director, Association for the Advancement of Automotive Medicine

Layout and Format: Irene Herzau

はじめに

人体への損傷をその形態と重症度によって適切に分類することは外傷の病因論の研究に必須である。損傷をカテゴリー化するためのスケールは2つのタイプに分類できる：1つは，患者の生理学的な状態を評価するスケールであり，受傷後の時間経過とともに変化する。もう1つは，解剖学的部位や損傷の局在，相対的な重症度で損傷を表現するものである。

1. AISの起源

1960年代，多角的な交通事故調査チームが組織されたのと時を同じくして，損傷形態と重症度についての標準化された分類法の必要性が生じた。この調査チームは，技術者，医者，解剖学者/生理学者，事故調査の専門家などから構成されていた。調査チームの目的は，車両の設計を人体損傷の発生頻度と発生機序から評価できるように疫学的なデータを提供することであった。American Medical Association (AMA), Association for the Advancement of Automotive Medicine (AAAM), およびSociety of Automotive Engineers (SAE) の後援を受け，これらの専門家を主体にした協議会によって，1971年[1]にAbbreviated Injury Scale (AIS) として発表された。AIS初版は，コーネル大学のDeHaven[2]による先駆的な業績や，世界中の研究者[3-9]によってそれまでに発表された各種のスケールを参考にして作成された。このAISはきわめて初歩的なものであったが，米運輸省はじめ，米国内，欧州，豪州の大学関連あるいは企業のさまざまな事故調査チームにとって損傷を記述するさいの標準となった。このような初期の損傷スケール化作業では，人体に対する損傷を的確に表現するためには他のパラメータを考慮することも必要であるという概念も導入された[10]。

その後，1973年にAISの運用主体はAAAMに移り，74年，75年に若干の修正[11,12]が行われ，76年には500項目の損傷コードを含む最初のAIS手引書が発刊された[13]。1980年には脳損傷，熱傷，皮膚損傷が組み入れられ，全体的な重症度評価についての損傷スケーリングの改変が行われAIS80としてまとめられた[14]。

AISは当初，鈍的外傷を評価するために開発されたものであるが，1980年代になり外傷治療システムの進歩と患者登録制度が発展すると，穿通性損傷についてもコード化する必要性が生じてきた。臨床的に使用できる「言語」として新たな損傷の記述法はAIS85に取り入れられた。ここには主に血管系と体表（皮膚）損傷に関する記述法が追加された。とくに胸部，腹部の損傷と重症度が拡充され，以前の版に比して確実な損傷コード選択が可能になった[15]。

AIS90ではシステム全体に大きな変更が加えられているが，特別な改良点については後述する。

2. AISの目的と概念

AISは，損傷を重症度によってランクづけして数値化することと，損傷を記述するための用語を標準化することを目的に発展してきた。1971年以来AISはこの目標に沿って，より洗練されるべく改良が加えられ，損傷内容をより詳しくコード化するだけでなく，損傷の記述法は自動車事故以外の損傷に対しても拡張された。AISは当初，基本的には大規模な自動車事故データに適合させたものであったが，版を重ねるに従い臨床医学研究の分野にも応用可能となり，外傷に関する調査研究のため世界中で利用されている。

AISは版を重ねるたびに変貌してきてはいるが，最初から受け継がれている3つの原則がある。これらの原則はAISの有用性を保持してきたと同時に限界をも明確にしてきた。

第一に，損傷の記述は解剖学的見地からのみ行い，生理学的見地によらないことである。すなわち，1つの損傷に対し，単一のAISコードのみが対応し，これは時間経過による損傷状態の生理学的変化に影響されないことである。これに対して，生理学的パラメータを用いるスケールの場合，時間による損傷状態の生理学的変化によってスコア自体が変化することになる。

第二に，AISは損傷それ自体をスコア化するものなので，損傷によって引き起こされた結果——機能障害——については考慮してこなかった。しかし，AISの発展につれて，特殊な損傷については損傷の重症度をより正確に記述するため，損傷に伴ってただちに起こる病態を考慮することにした。例えば，脳損傷による意識障害，血管損傷や実質臓器損傷による出血，胸部外傷による気胸などである。

第三に，AISは予測される死亡率に基づいて単純にランクづけしたものではないことである。もしそうであるならば，ほとんどの軽症，中等症は生命の危険がないのでこれらを区別してスコア化することができなくなる。AISが3以上の損傷（重症ないし重篤）については，経験的にAIS自体が死亡率と相関することが判明しているが，AISの重症度においては他の因子も取り入れている。すなわち，生命への危険性，診断の確かさ，病態の進行速度と持続時間，損傷の複雑性，治療の有効性などの因子である。これらの因子は定量化するのは困難だが，重症度というものは医学の進歩により継続的に再定義されるべきものと思われるので，損傷程度を記述するさいに考慮すべきである。

AISはこれら3つの原則を保ちながら今後も改良していく予定である。

3．多発外傷の評価

AISは，解剖学的な身体部位ごとにそれぞれの損傷を分類し，重症度をAIS 1（軽症）からAIS 6（救命不能）までの6段階で評価するシステムである。AIS自体は多発外傷における複合重症度を評価するわけではない。

多発外傷では最大AIS（MAIS：各部位のAISのうち最大のもの）を総合的な重症度とする考え方があり，自動車の衝突安全設計を考える研究者たちに支持されている。しかし外傷においては，MAISは生命の危険度と比例しないことがわかっている。MAISが同一でも2番目に大きいAISに影響され死亡率が変化することが知られているからである。

1974年にBakerによって発表されたInjury Severity Score（ISS）は，身体各部位の最大AISのうち，上位3部位の値の自乗和として定義され，このスコアによる重症度は死亡率とよく相関している[16,17]（ISSの計算方法は21，22ページ参照）。

4．ICDとAISの互換性

ICDコードとAISコード間の変換表がMacKenzieにより1986年に発表された[18]。損傷の最終診断名をICD-9 CM方式によりコード化したものをAISの損傷部位と重症度に変換するものである。AIS85では，多くの損傷名がICDの見出しに一致していたため，ICDからAIS85への変換が可能であった。ICDからAIS90へ変換可能であるかどうかは検討中である（AIS90を基にした改訂版がある）。

AIS90における改良点

AIS90は，約20年間にわたる臨床応用と研究分野での成果に基づいて改良された。以下，その改良点について簡潔に述べる。

1．コード選択のガイドライン

損傷データを収集するときの問題は，(1)損傷スケール自体に関すること，(2)コード選択者にとって情報が限られていること，(3)コード選択者の資質に影響されること，などである。AISコードは初版の75項目から，鈍的損傷と穿通性損傷に適合した1300項目へと拡張され，用語も標準化されたので以前よりもコード選択がしやすくなった。さらに，AISの利用者に対しては，コードの選択方法に関するトレーニングセミナーをAAAMが開催している。

損傷に関する情報が不十分であるときは，AISコード自体やコード選択者自身の資質に関するよりも問題が大きい。例えば，「多発性鈍的損傷により死に至った」という剖検報告は，損傷についての何ら特別な情報を与えていないので，損傷のコードを選択する目的には実際上利用できない。病院診療録でさえ詳細に至っては欠落が多いこともあるし，記録の一部に損傷情報の矛盾があることもある。

AIS90の手引書は，損傷部位および損傷形態の選択を容易にできるように特別なルールに従って作成されている。たとえば同義語，カッコ付きの用語を用いることにより診療録に記載された臨床診断名から適切なコードが選択できるように配慮されている。コード選択者が訓練を積めば再現性と信頼性を高めるのに役立つ。

2．穿通性損傷

AIS85において初めて銃創や刺創などの穿通性損傷もコード化の対象となった。さらに血管系，胸部および腹部臓器の穿通性損傷に臨床的に使用されている用語もAIS85に採用された。その経験がAISにおける用語の改良につながり，AIS90では，穿通性損傷の記述法はすべての部位で一致したものとなった。血管損傷のAISコードは最近数年間における臨床研究，とくに全米規模で行われた重症外傷予後調査 Major Trauma Outcome Study（MTOS）[19]の成果を反映させた。

3．小児外傷

損傷の重症度は年齢により大きく影響される。損傷程度が同じ場合，高齢者では若年者よりも予後が悪いことが知られており，幼児の場合も高齢者と同様の傾向をもつと思われる。

数年前Bakerは，小児外傷外科医を招集し，AIS85におけるすべての損傷項目とそれらの重症度について小児外傷に適応できない項目があるかどうかを再調査した。その結果，1300以上の損傷項目のうち15項目を除くすべての項目が，小児においても相対的には重症度を反映しているとの意見の一致をみた。例外となった15の損傷とは，脳の血腫の大きさ，重症裂創における出血量，胸腹部損傷における胸腔，腹腔内の出血量に関係するものであった。損傷スケーリング委員会は，一部はすべての年齢に適用し得るとしたものの，小

児外傷における数値の変更に関する提言に同意し，これらの修正はAIS90に組み込まれている。

4．損傷リストの拡張

AISは機能障害，後遺障害については評価していない。AISを補完し，重症度と社会的費用を関連づける尺度をもつことはきわめて重要なことであり，すでに数種のスケールが考案されている[20-22]。

最近States[23]によって提言された機能障害スケールの構想が，AAAMの損傷スケーリング委員会で取り上げられ，診断基準が審議されている。将来の新しいスケールを念頭において，AISの損傷リストは機能障害がコード化に対応できるように拡張されている。損傷を受けた臓器の種類により，AISが同一でも機能障害程度はそれぞれ異なるのが普通であるが，障害をスケール化するためには，さらに正確な損傷診断が必要とされる。

5．損傷コードの見方

AIS85は，コンピュータ処理のために各損傷を6桁の数値（コード）で表現していた。AIS90では，損傷の記述法が拡張されたため（とくに脳と四肢），より柔軟な数値化システムが必要となった。

AIS90では，損傷部位と損傷形態を表す6桁の数値と，重症度スコアを表す1桁の数値によって損傷コードが構成されている。右ページの図に示すように左から1桁目は損傷区分，2桁目は解剖学上の構造，3および4桁目は損傷分類の名称，5および6桁目は各部位における損傷レベルにそれぞれ対応し，小数点の右側はAISスコアである。

6．体表損傷

AIS90以前は，皮膚ないし体表損傷は，身体のどの部位にあっても「体表」の項目（External section）に分類していたが，それでは車両設計または事故対策（例えば，シートベルト装着を義務づける条例が顔面外傷を減らす効果があったかどうか）の目的でAISを利用するさいに，損傷部位が特定できないという問題が生じた。AISが2以下の顔面外傷は体表の区分に分類されたため，部位が顔面であることがわからなかったのである。

AIS90では，体表損傷（皮膚，皮下組織，筋などを含む）はその身体部位が容易に特定できるように，身体部位ごとにコードをもつようにした。ただし，この変更によって，損傷を「体表」を含む身体6部位に分類しているISS（Injury Severity Score）を計算するさいに問題が生じる可能性がでてきた。そこで，全体的な重症度評価に影響を与えぬように，体表損傷を伴うときにはISSの計算に当たって特別のルールが決められている(21ページ参照)。

7．脳損傷

AISが3以上の脳損傷は他の部位の損傷に比較して過小評価されているとする損傷スケール委員会の結論は，MTOSのような大規模データベースの解析結果によっても支持された[24]。

これを改善するためAIS90では，「脳」の章は大幅に拡張され，脳挫傷はその範囲，局在部位，および単発性か多発性かによってAIS3～5のコードに分類された。大脳および小脳血腫の量，大きさ，局在についても

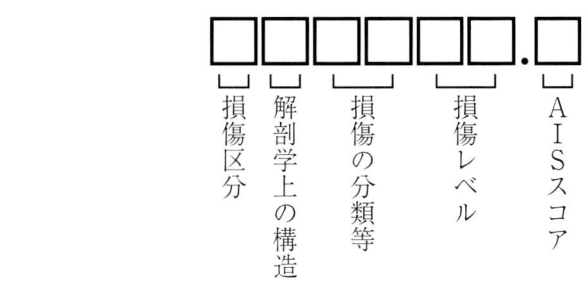

以下は，損傷を数値化するさいの規則である。

1桁目：損傷区分
1　頭部
2　顔面
3　頸部
4　胸部
5　腹部
6　脊椎
7　上肢
8　下肢
9　その他

2桁目：解剖学上の構造
1　全域
2　血管
3　神経
4　内臓（筋・靱帯を含む）
5　骨格（関節を含む）
6　頭部－意識障害

3－4桁目：解剖学上の部位もしくは損傷の種類

全域
- 02　皮膚 － 擦過傷（Abrasion）
- 04　　　 － 挫傷（Contusion）
- 06　　　 － 裂創（Laceration）
- 08　　　 － 剥離（Avulsion）
- 10　切断（Amputation）
- 20　熱傷（Burn）
- 30　挫滅（Crush）
- 40　デグロービング損傷（Degloving）
- 50　詳細不明（NFS：Not Further Specified）
- 60　穿通性損傷（Penetrating）
- 09　機械的外力以外による損傷（Trauma, other than mechanical）

頭部－意識障害
- 02　意識障害（LOC）の持続時間
- 04，06，08　意識レベル
- 10　脳震盪（Concussion）

脊椎
- 02　頸椎
- 04　胸椎
- 06　腰椎

血管，神経，臓器，骨格および関節
　個々の部位に02に続く2桁の数値を当てる

5－6桁目：損傷程度（Level）
- ・個々の損傷には02に続く2桁の数値を当てる。
- ・00は損傷程度が詳細不明であることを示す。
- ・99は損傷形態が詳細不明であることを示す。

実際の重症度を反映するように再評価され，これらの損傷を記述する用語は臨床的にも許容できるものになっている。また，「血管，頭蓋内」と「脳神経」の2つの章を追加した。

8．用語の修正と変更

　AIS90では頸部，胸部，腹部における血管損傷を明確にするため，用語と重症度の両面にわたって変更がなされた。また，腹部臓器損傷の記述法，用語の修正が行われ，現在，臨床と外傷研究とで使われている損傷分類との整合性をもたせた。この改善はとくに穿通性損傷のコード選択に役立つだろう。

　また，深部の損傷を伴わない穿通性損傷と体表面の裂創についての用語も変更された。

ま と め

　AIS は当初，自動車事故に関連した損傷の発生頻度と重症度を標準化するために開発されたものである。その利用範囲は疫学的調査研究，外傷センターにおける生存予測の研究，外傷患者の予後評価，健康管理の研究にも拡張され，さらには外傷治療における社会的費用の評価研究にも利用されてきた。

　AIS は ISS 算出の基礎となっており，将来的にも，損傷重症度を評価するための基本システムであり続けるだろう。AIS は世界標準であり，外傷データを適切に収集するためには，これを正確に継続して使用することが必須である。

References

1. Rating the severity of tissue damage: I. The Abbreviated Injury Scale, JAMA 215 : 277-280, 1971.
2. DeHaven H, The site, frequency and dangerousness of injury sustained by 800 survivors of light plane accidents. Crash Injury Research, Department of Public Health and Preventive Medicine, Cornell University Medical College, New York, July 1952.
3. Ryan GA and Garrett JW, A Quantitative Scale of Impact Injury, publication CAL No. VT 1823-R34, Cornell Aeronautical Laboratory, Inc., Buffalo, New York, October 1968.
4. Mackay GM, Road Accident Research Project Report No. 4, Human Engineering Section, Department of Transportation and Environmental Planning, University of Birmingham, England, December 1966.
5. Williams RE and Schamadan JL, The "Simbol" Rating and Evaluation System, ARIZONA MEDICINE 26 : 886-887, 1969.
6. Campbell EO, Collision Tissue Damage Record, Traffic Injury Research Foundation, Ottawa, Canada, 1966.
7. States JD, Scale developed by Research Accident Investigation Team, University of Rochester School of Medicine, New York, 1969.
8. Nahum A, Siegel AW and Hight PV, Injuries to rear seat occupants in automobile collisions, Proceedings, 11th Stapp Car Crash Conference, New York (Society of Automotive Engneers, Warrendale, PA, 1967).
9. Huelke DF, University of Michigan Multidisciplinary Accident Investigation Team, Ann Arbor, MI, 1968.
10. States JD, The Abbreviated and the Comprehensive Research Injury Scales, STAPP Proceedings, 13 : 282-294, (SAE 690810) 1969.
11. States JD, Huelke DF, Hames LN, 1974 AMA-SAE-AAAM revision of the Abbreviated Injury Scale (AIS), AAAM Proceedings 18 : 479-505.
12. Joint Committee on Injury Scaling of SAE-AAAM-AMA, The Abbreviated Injury Scale (1975 revision), AAAM Proceedings 19 : 438-466.
13. The Abbreviated Injury Scale (AIS) 1976 revision, including Dictionary, American Association for Automotive Medicine (now Association for the Advancement of Automotive Medicine), Des Plaines, IL.
14. The Abbreviated Injury Scale 1980 Revision, American Association for Automotive Medicine (now Association for the Advancement of Automotive Medicine), Des Plaines, IL.
15. The Abbreviated Injury Scale 1985 Revision, American Association for Automotive Medicine (now Association for the Advancement of Automotive Medicine), Des Plaines, IL.
16. Baker SP, O'Neill B, Haddon W, Long WB, The Injury Severity Score: A method for describing patients with multiple injuries and evaluating emergency care. J Trauma 14 : 187-196, 1974.
17. Bull JP, The Injury Severity Score of road traffic casualties in relation to mortality, time of death, hospital treatment time and disability, Accid Anal & Prev 7 : 249-255, 1975.
18. MacKenzie EJ, Steinwachs DM, Shankar BS, Classifying severity of trauma based on hospital discharge diagnosis: Validation of an ICD-9CM to AIS-85 conversion table, Medical Care 27 : 412-422, 1989.
19. Champion HR, Copes WS, Sacco WJ, Major Trauma Outcome Study: Establishing national norms for trauma care, J Trauma 30 : 1356-1365, 1990.
20. Hirsch AE, Eppinger RH, Impairment scaling from the Abbreviated Injury Scale, AAAM Proceedings 28 : 209-224, 1984.
21. Gustafsson H, Nygren A, Tingvall C, Permanent medical impairment among road traffic victims and risk of serious consequences, RSC, SAE International Congress and Exposition, 1986.
22. The Development of an Impairment Index for Traumatic Injuries, in progress at Johns Hopkins University, Baltimore, MD.
23. States JD and Viano DC, Injury impairment and disability scales to assess the permanent consequences of trauma, Acc Anal & Prev 22 : 151-160, April 1990.
24. Gennarelli TA, Champion HR, Sacco WJ, Copes WS and Alves WM, Mortality of patients with head injury and extracranial injury treated in trauma centers, J Trauma 29 : 1193-1202, September 1989.

手引書の使い方

1. 様　式

　AISの手引書は，人体を次の9つに「区分」して記述されている。「頭部」「顔面」「頸部」「胸部」「腹部および骨盤内臓器」「脊椎」「上肢」「下肢」「体表およびその他」である。これらの「区分」は後述するISSの計算で適用する6つの「部位」とは異なる。そのため，ISSを計算するときはAISの「区分」とISSの「部位」を間違わないように注意しなければならない。

　脊椎，体表，熱傷およびその他の外傷を除いて，それぞれの部位における損傷内容は全域，血管，神経，内臓，骨格の順に分類され，損傷部の解剖学的名称のアルファベット順に並んでいる。上肢および下肢については，筋肉，腱，靱帯の項目がある。ほとんどの場合，損傷内容は軽度なものから重症度の順に並んでいる。

　本書の索引にはAIS90に収載されている損傷内容の全リストがアルファベット順に記載され，前述のAIS90の9つの「区分」と記載ページが併記されている。

　それぞれの損傷には7桁の数値（コード）が決められている（12, 13ページ参照）。小数点以下は重症度で，下記に示すとおりである。

AISコードの重症度	内　容
1	軽　症 (Minor)
2	中等症 (Moderate)
3	重　症 (Serious)
4	重　篤 (Severe)
5	瀕　死 (Critical)
6	救命不能 (Maximum)

2. コード選択のルール

　この手引書には，コード選択に関する2種類の注釈がある。第一はカッコ内に書かれた注釈である。これは損傷内容の同義語あるいは詳細な情報で，診療録などに記載されている情報から適切なAISコードを選択できるように手助けするものである。第二は四角の枠内に太文字で表記されている注意書きで，適切なコードを選択するための補足的説明である。

　これらの注釈に加えて，以下のコード選択のルールをすべての損傷部位に適用する。これらのコード選択のルールを熟知し，例外なく適用し均一なコード選択を図るべきである。

1．あらゆる情報をもとにしても損傷程度が明確でなければ，控えめにコードを選択しなければならない（すなわち，その損傷に対応する AIS コードが複数考えられた場合は重症度がもっとも低い AIS コードを選択する）。

2．AIS6は重症度が6に決められた特定の損傷についてのみ適用すること。AIS6は，患者が死亡したからといって，その結果だけで単純に選択してはいけない。AIS5の損傷がAIS6に上がることは決してない。

3．診療録に記載された疑い病名（疑診）は，医学的に証明されていなければコード選択の対象とすべきではない。

4．AIS のコード選択の対象は損傷の結果生じる障害（例えば失明）ではなく，その原因となった損傷（例えば視神経の離断）である。

5．異物は損傷でないためコード選択の対象にならない。

6．外科的手技あるいはその他の処置などを参考にして損傷の重症度を判断すべきではない。処置だけを根拠にして損傷の重症度を高くしてはいけない。（訳注：例えば，診療録に胸腔ドレナージを行った記載があっても，それだけで血気胸があるとは判断できない）

7．腎臓，眼，耳や四肢など対をなす臓器の両側に損傷がある場合は，それぞれ別々にコードを選択しなければならない。ただし，上顎骨，下顎骨，骨盤，胸郭および肺は単一の臓器としてコードを選択する。

8．開放骨折とは，骨折部位に皮膚裂創を伴う骨折と定義する。開放骨折の裂創は自動的に骨折のコードに含まれており，あらためてコード選択しない。

9．厳密に言えば，「挫滅（crush）」は受傷原因を示す用語である。しかし，この語は診療録やその他の記録（訳注：剖検記録など）に使われているため，AISでも使用されている。コード選択の目的で用いる「挫滅」とは骨格，血管，軟部組織系の破壊を意味する重篤な損傷である。「挫滅」は，その損傷が本手引き書の基準に合致する場合のみ適用する。「挫滅」をコード選択した場合，同一区分の個々の損傷をコード選択してはならない。（訳注：個々の損傷をコード選択できる場合は「挫滅」を選択しない）

10．血管の損傷が「断裂」と記載されている場合，完全な切断としてコード選択する。「不完全」断裂と記載されている場合，「断裂」よりも重症度が低いコードを選択する。例えば，大動脈断裂は520208.5で

あり，不完全断裂は520206.4である。

11. 胸部の区分に複数の損傷を認め，血気胸，縦隔血腫，縦隔気腫を伴う場合，これらの病態を含むコードは1つしか選択できない。（訳注：例えば，縦隔血腫を伴う大動脈損傷420216.5と縦隔血腫を伴う肺裂傷441418.4を同時に選択することはできない）。

12. 複数の損傷に「出血量20％を超える」というコードが該当する場合，出血にもっとも関与したと思われる損傷にのみこのコードを選択する。

13. 出血量の推定――一般的に診療録には，出血量が全血液量に対する比率で記載されていない。次の表を用いることで全血液の20％に相当する出血量を推定できる。この表は小児の場合にも使用できる。大まかに言って，1000mlは平均成人の全血液量の20％に相当する。

体重	20％の出血量
kg	ml
100	1500
75	1125
50	750
25	375
10	150
5	75

14. 臓器損傷に血管損傷が伴う場合，それが当該臓器の損傷内容に記述されていれば，血管損傷を独立してコード選択しない。したがって，以下に示す50ページの例では，腎血管損傷をコード選択しない。

例 　　　　　　　　　　　　　　　　　　　　AISコード
腎皮質を貫通し，髄質，腎盂腎杯に達する損傷；　541626.4
腎茎部の血管損傷で出血を伴う

15. 穿通性損傷のコード選択を行うとき，深部の組織損傷を選択し，体表損傷のコードを選択しない。出入口部の体表損傷は臓器損傷の重症度に含まれる。

例 　　　　　　　　　　　　　　AISコード
肝臓に対する銃創，出血量が　　　541824.3
全血液量の20％を超える

例外1：穿通性損傷の部位しかわからない場合

例	AIS コード
腹部に対する銃創	516000.1
あるいは	
出血量が1000mlを超える腹部に対する銃創	516006.3

例外2：脳に対する穿通性損傷が複数領域にわたる場合（例えば，大脳から入って小脳へ抜ける穿通性損傷）は，脳の特定部位ではなく「全域」に分類されている116004.5「深い穿通性損傷」を使用する。

例外3：穿通性損傷のコード選択により，個々の臓器損傷を選択するより重症度が高くなる場合

例	AIS コード
頭部銃創で以下の損傷があるとき；これらの3つのコードを選択するのではなく，穿通性損傷（大脳）140690.5のコードを選択する。	
小さな硬膜下血腫	140652.4
くも膜下出血	140684.3
軽症脳腫脹	140662.3

情報が欠如している場合や，上記3つの例外を網羅するために，脊椎を除く各章の「全域」には「穿通性損傷」のコードがある。

16．「損傷程度が不明な損傷」とは，損傷形態（例えば裂創）はわかっているが，その損傷程度が特定できないあるいは不明確な損傷をいう。この場合，「裂創　詳細不明」としてコード選択する。コード00（訳注：整数部分の下2桁が"00"であるコード）は多くの場合，損傷程度がわからない損傷のコードになっている（12ページ「5．損傷コードの見方」を参照）。

17．「損傷形態が不明な損傷」とは損傷の生じている部位や臓器はわかるが，詳細な損傷形態のわからない損傷をいう。例えば，「腎損傷」と記載されていれば腎の挫傷あるいは裂傷（裂創）であると類推できるが，これだけでは損傷形態が不明確である。この例において，腎損傷は「詳細不明」としてコード選択される。コード99（訳注：整数部分の下2桁が"99"であるコード）は損傷形態あるいは損傷程度がわからない損傷のコードである（12ページ「5．損傷コードの見方」を参照）。
（訳注：16，17のルールに従えば「詳細不明」としてコード選択された損傷でもISSは計算することができる）

18．あいまいな記述しかない場合
「鈍的外傷」や「閉鎖性頭部損傷」のようなあいまいな記述はいまだに使われているが，確定的な診断ではないため正確なAISコードを選択できない。これが唯一の記述であれば，「詳細不明 NFS（not further

specified)」の AIS コードを選択する。このようなコードは，手引書の各区分に含まれている（例えば，閉鎖性頭部損傷　詳細不明，鈍的腹部損傷）。このようなあいまいな記述でも外傷の発生頻度を調査するときには利用することができる。しかし，前述のようなあいまいな記述のために「詳細不明」とコード選択された損傷は ISS の計算に使うことができない。

3．ISS（Injury Severity Score）の計算

A．一般的なルール

ISS は，6 部位の AIS スコアの中から，上位 3 つを自乗して合計した値である。ISS の 6 部位は次のとおりである。

> 1. 頭頸部
> 2. 顔面
> 3. 胸部
> 4. 腹部および骨盤内臓器
> 5. 四肢および骨盤
> 6. 体表
>
> 「頭頸部」には，脳，頸髄の損傷，頭蓋骨，頸椎の骨折を含む。
> 「顔面」には，口，耳，眼，鼻および顔面骨の損傷を含む。
> 「胸部」「腹部および骨盤内臓器」には，それぞれ，胸腔，腹腔および骨盤内のすべての臓器損傷を含む。また，「胸部」には，横隔膜，胸郭，胸椎の損傷を含む。腰椎の損傷は，「腹部および骨盤内臓器」に含まれる。
> 「四肢および骨盤」には，脊椎，頭蓋骨および肋骨以外の捻挫，骨折，脱臼，切断を含む。
> 「体表」には，裂創，挫傷，擦過傷あるいは熱傷を含み，その部位には関係しない。

なお，ISS の「部位」は，AIS の「区分」とは必ずしも一致しない。例えば，脊椎損傷は ISS では 3 つの「部位」に分けられる。例えば，頸椎は ISS の「部位」では「頭頸部」に，同様に胸椎は「胸部」に，腰椎は「腹部および骨盤内臓器」に分類される。

次の例が ISS 計算の一例である。

ISSでの部位	損　　傷	AISコード	最大AIS	AIS²
頭頸部	脳挫傷 頸動脈の完全断裂	140604.3 320212.4	4	16
顔面	耳裂創	210600.1	1	
胸部	肋骨骨折 左側第3〜第4肋骨	450220.2	2	
腹部	後腹膜血腫	543800.3	3	9
四肢	大腿骨骨折	851800.3	3	9
体表	全身の擦過傷	910200.1	1	
				(ISS＝34)

　ISSは1〜75の範囲である。ISSが75となるのは，AIS5の損傷が3つ，あるいはAIS6の損傷が少なくとも1つある場合のどちらかである。AIS6のコードが選択された損傷がある場合，ISSは自動的に75となる。ISSが75の場合，他の損傷を加えてもISSは増えないが，すべての損傷のコードを選択しなくてはならない。小数点以下が9であるAISコードを選択した場合は，ISSを計算することはできない。したがって，ISSを計算できるよう損傷を詳細に記述すべきである。

B．皮膚損傷のコード選択

　AIS90より前は，皮膚の損傷や穿通性損傷については，体表の「区分」でコードを選択し，ISSの計算でも体表の部位で計算されていた。AISでは皮膚の損傷に対して，その損傷が存在する「区分」ごとにコードを定め，皮膚の損傷をより正確に記述できるようになった（12ページ「6．体表損傷」を参照）。この変更は，総合的な重症度評価（訳注：ISSの計算）に影響しない。

　体表損傷を伴う場合のISSの計算のルールは次のとおりである。

　1．体表損傷が単独に生じた場合（すなわち，臓器の損傷がない場合）は，適切なAISの「区分」でコード選択する（例えば，顎裂創210600.1）。ただし，ISSの計算では体表として計算する。

　2．多数のAIS1の体表損傷が複数の区分にわたって生じた場合（すなわち，全身の擦過傷および挫傷，詳細不明），体表(73ページ参照)でコード選択してもよい（すなわち，擦過傷910200.1，挫傷910400.1）。また，ISSの計算では一括して体表として計算する。

　3．体表損傷が深部組織の損傷を伴っている場合，両損傷ともコードを選択する（例えば，胸壁挫傷410402.1，肺挫傷441406.3）。ISSの計算では，皮膚の損傷は「体表」で計算し，胸腔内臓器の損傷は「胸部」で計算する。このルールの例外は，開放骨折（18ページの第8項）と穿通性損傷（19ページの第15項）である。

頭　部
（頭蓋と脳）

HEAD (cranium and brain)

CODE	INJURY DESCRIPTION

WHOLE AREA

113000.6   Massive destruction of both cranium (skull) and brain (**Crush**)

> Code penetrating injuries to cerebrum, cerebellum or brainstem if specific location is known, and do not therefore use this section in those circumstances. Use one of the following two descriptions only if (1) specific site is unknown or (2) the "penetrating injury" description results in a higher AIS code than the specific anatomically described injury.

Penetrating injury   if no skull penetration or NFS, code as scalp laceration

116002.3   superficial (≤2cm beneath entrance)
116004.5   major (>2cm penetration)

> Assign one of the following codes, as appropriate, to soft tissue (external or subgaleal) injuries to the scalp. To calculate an ISS, however, assign injuries in this category to the External body region and follow rules for ISS calculation on pages xviii and xix.

110099.1   **Scalp** NFS
110202.1   abrasion
110402.1   contusion (includes subgaleal hematoma)
110600.1   laceration NFS
110602.1   minor, superficial
110604.2   major (>10cm long and into subcutaneous tissue)
110606.3   blood loss >20% by volume
110800.1   avulsion NFS
110802.1   superficial; minor (≤100cm^2)
110804.2   major (>100cm^2 but blood loss <20% by volume)
110806.3   blood loss >20% by volume
110808.3   total scalp loss

> Use one of the following two descriptors when such vague information is the only description available. These descriptors allow a means of identifying the occurrence of head injury, but they do not allow the calculation of an accurate ISS in these patients.

115099.9   **Closed head injury** NFS   Use also for traumatic brain injury NFS
115999.9   Died without further evaluation; no autopsy.

頭部（頭蓋と脳）

| コード | 損傷内容 |

全 域

113000.6　頭蓋（骨）および脳の広範囲損傷（挫滅）

> 大脳，小脳あるいは脳幹の穿通性損傷で損傷部位が特定できている場合は，以下の穿通性損傷のコードを選択せずに，該当する各々に対する穿通性損傷のコードを選択する。以下の穿通性損傷のコードは次の2つのうちいずれか1つが当てはまる場合にのみ選択する：(1)損傷部位を特定できない，あるいは(2)"穿通性損傷"としたAISコード点数の方が他の損傷を解剖学的に特定したAISコード点数よりも高くなる場合。

穿通性損傷　骨を穿通していない場合，詳細不明の場合は「頭皮裂創」のコードを選択する。

116002.3　　　　表在性（創の深さが2 cm以下）
116004.5　　　　深い（創の深さが2 cmを超える）

> 頭皮の軟部組織（皮膚あるいは帽状腱膜下）の損傷には，以下の適切なコードを割り当てる。ただしISSを算出する場合には，「頭部」ではなく「体表」の区分として取り扱い，21，22ページのISS計算ルールに従う。

110099.1　**頭皮**　詳細不明
110202.1　　　擦過傷
110402.1　　　挫傷（帽状腱膜下血腫を含む）
110600.1　　　裂創　詳細不明
110602.1　　　　　小；表在性
110604.2　　　　　大；（長さが10cmを超え，かつ皮下組織まで達している）
110606.3　　　　　出血量が全血液量の20％を超える
110800.1　　　剝離　詳細不明
110802.1　　　　　表在性；小（100cm²以下）
110804.2　　　　　大（100cm²を超えるが，出血量は全血液量の20％以下）
110806.3　　　　　出血量が全血液量の20％を超える
110808.3　　　　　全頭皮剝脱

> 不確定な情報しか得られない場合には，以下の2つのコードのうちいずれかを選択する。ただしこれらのコードを選択した場合にISSは計算してはならない。

115099.9　**閉鎖性頭部損傷**　詳細不明　詳細不明の外傷性脳損傷にも使用する。
115999.9　　　死亡（詳細な評価なし）；剖検なし

HEAD (cranium and brain)

CODE	INJURY DESCRIPTION

VESSELS, INTRACRANIAL

> The following major vessel injuries should be coded separate from the injuries to the brain. If specific major vessel is not known, code as intracranial vessel NFS, 121299.3.
>
> Thrombosis includes any injury to the vessel resulting in its occlusion (e. g., intimal tear, dissection).

120299.3	**Anterior cerebral artery** NFS
120202.5	laceration
120204.3	thrombosis (occlusion)
120206.3	traumatic aneurysm
120499.5	**Basilar artery** NFS
120402.5	laceration
120404.5	thrombosis (occlusion)
120406.5	traumatic aneurysm
120602.4	**Carotid-cavernous** fistula
120899.3	**Cavernous sinus** NFS
120802.4	laceration
120804.5	open laceration or segmental loss ("open" means vessel is bleeding out of the body externally.)
120806.3	thrombosis (occlusion)
121099.3	**Internal carotid artery** NFS
121002.5	laceration
121004.4	thrombosis (occlusion)
121006.3	traumatic aneurysm
121299.3	**Intracranial vessel** NFS Use this description if specific vessel is not known.
121202.4	laceration
121204.3	thrombosis (occlusion)
121206.3	traumatic aneurysm
121499.3	**Middle cerebral artery** NFS
121402.5	laceration
121404.4	thrombosis (occlusion)
121406.3	traumatic aneurysm
121699.3	**Other artery** NFS (branch of anterior, posterior or middle cerebral artery or branches of basilar or vertebral artery)
121602.4	laceration
121604.3	thrombosis (occlusion)
121606.3	traumatic aneurysm

コード	損傷内容

血管，頭蓋内

> 以下の主要血管損傷は脳損傷とは別個にコードを選択する。どの主要血管か特定できない場合は頭蓋内血管 詳細不明(121299.3)のコードを選択する。
>
> 血栓症は，血管の閉塞をまねく血管損傷をすべて含む（例；動脈内膜損傷，解離など）。

120299.3	前大脳動脈	詳細不明
120202.5		裂傷
120204.3		血栓症（閉塞）
120206.3		外傷性動脈瘤
120499.5	脳底動脈	詳細不明
120402.5		裂傷
120404.5		血栓症（閉塞）
120406.5		外傷性動脈瘤
120602.4	頸動脈-海綿静脈洞瘻	
120899.3	海綿静脈洞	詳細不明
120802.4		裂傷
120804.5		開放性裂傷または部分欠損（"開放性"は，その血管から体外に出血していることを意味する）
120806.3		血栓症（閉塞）
121099.3	内頸動脈	詳細不明
121002.5		裂傷
121004.4		血栓症（閉塞）
121006.3		外傷性動脈瘤
121299.3	頭蓋内血管	詳細不明 　　どの血管か特定されていない場合は，このコードを選択する。
121202.4		裂傷
121204.3		血栓症（閉塞）
121206.3		外傷性動脈瘤
121499.3	中大脳動脈	詳細不明
121402.5		裂傷
121404.4		血栓症（閉塞）
121406.3		外傷性動脈瘤
121699.3	その他の動脈（前，中，後大脳動脈，脳底動脈，椎骨動脈の各分枝）詳細不明	
121602.4		裂傷
121604.3		血栓症（閉塞）
121606.3		外傷性動脈瘤

HEAD (cranium and brain)

CODE	INJURY DESCRIPTION

121899.3	**Posterior cerebral artery** NFS
121802.5	laceration
121804.3	thrombosis (occlusion)
121806.3	traumatic aneurysm

122099.4	**Sigmoid sinus** NFS
122002.4	laceration
122004.5	open laceration or segmental loss ("open" means vessel is bleeding outside the body externally.)
122006.4	thrombosis (occlusion)

122299.3	**Sinus** NFS or **major vein** NFS
122202.4	laceration
122204.3	thrombosis (occlusion)

122499.4	**Superior longitudinal (sagittal) sinus** NFS
122402.4	laceration
122404.5	open laceration or segmental loss ("open" means vessel is bleeding outside the body externally.)
122406.4	thrombosis (occlusion)

122699.4	**Transverse sinus** NFS
122602.4	laceration
122604.5	open laceration or segmental loss ("open" means vessel is bleeding outside the body externally.)
122606.4	thrombosis (occlusion)

122899.3	**Vertebral artery** NFS
122802.5	laceration
122804.3	thrombosis (occlusion)
122806.3	traumatic aneurysm

NERVES, CRANIAL

> Because of limitations in diagnostic capabilities, it is often impossible to assign specific injury descriptors to cranial nerve injuries. Therefore, many cranial nerve injuries may be described only by the type of dysfunction that exists in normal nerve function. Unless contusion or laceration is specified, code as laceration if total loss of nerve function (paralysis) is described. Code as contusion if subtotal loss of function (paresis) is documented. Do not increase the severity for bilateral or multiple injuries of the same nerve. Nerve injuries should be coded separate from the injuries to the brain. If specific nerve is not known, code as cranial nerve NFS, code 130299.2.

130299.2	**Cranial nerve** NFS Use this description if specific nerve is not known.
130202.2	contusion
130204.2	laceration

130499.2	**I (Olfactory nerve, tract)** NFS
130402.2	contusion
130404.2	laceration

コード	損傷内容

121899.3　**後大脳動脈**　詳細不明
121802.5　　　　　裂傷
121804.3　　　　　血栓症（閉塞）
121806.3　　　　　外傷性動脈瘤

122099.4　**S状静脈洞**　詳細不明
122002.4　　　　　裂傷
122004.5　　　　　　　開放性裂傷または部分欠損（"開放性"は，その血管から体外に出血していることを意味する）
122006.4　　　　　血栓症（閉塞）

122299.3　**静脈洞または主要静脈**　詳細不明
122202.4　　　　　裂傷
122204.3　　　　　血栓症（閉塞）

122499.4　**上矢状洞**　詳細不明
122402.4　　　　　裂傷
122404.5　　　　　　　開放性裂傷または部分欠損（"開放性"は，その血管から体外に出血していることを意味する）
122406.4　　　　　血栓症（閉塞）

122699.4　**横静脈洞**　詳細不明
122602.4　　　　　裂傷
122604.5　　　　　　　開放性裂傷または部分欠損（"開放性"は，その血管から体外に出血していることを意味する）
122606.4　　　　　血栓症（閉塞）

122899.3　**椎骨動脈**　詳細不明
122802.5　　　　　裂傷
122804.3　　　　　血栓症（閉塞）
122806.3　　　　　外傷性動脈瘤

脳神経

> 脳神経損傷は，診断上の限界があるので損傷内容を解剖学的に特定することが不可能な場合もある。したがって脳神経損傷は，正常な神経機能に対する機能障害のタイプによってしか表現できないことも多い。挫傷，裂傷の特定ができない場合でも，神経機能の完全な消失（麻痺）が認められれば裂傷としてコードを選択する。また，神経機能の不完全な消失（不全麻痺）が認められる場合は挫傷としてコードを選択する。なお，同一の神経に生じた両側性もしくは多発性の損傷があっても重症度は変わらない。また，脳神経損傷は脳損傷とは別個にコードを選択する。もしどの脳神経か特定できない場合は，脳神経　詳細不明（130299.2）のコードを選択する。

130299.2　**脳神経**　詳細不明　　損傷した脳神経が特定できない場合にこのコードを選択する。
130202.2　　　　　挫傷
130204.2　　　　　裂傷

130499.2　**I（嗅神経，嗅神経路）**　詳細不明
130402.2　　　　　挫傷
130404.2　　　　　裂傷

HEAD (cranium and brain)

CODE	INJURY DESCRIPTION

130699.2   II (Optic nerve-intracranial and intracanalicular segments) NFS

> Code under Face section for intraorbital segment. If location is unknown, code under Head.

130602.2   contusion
130604.2   bilateral
130606.2   laceration
130608.2   bilateral

130899.2   III (Oculomotor nerve) NFS
130802.2   contusion or compression (includes injury due to transtentorial herniation)
130804.2   laceration

131099.2   IV (Trochlear nerve) NFS
131002.2   contusion
131004.2   laceration

131299.2   V (Trigeminal nerve) NFS
131202.2   contusion
131204.2   laceration

131499.2   VI (Abducens nerve) NFS
131402.2   contusion
131404.2   laceration

131699.2   VII (Facial nerve) NFS
131602.2   contusion
131604.2   laceration

131899.2   VIII (Acoustic Nerve, including auditory and vestibular nerves) NFS
131802.2   contusion
131804.2   laceration
131806.2   bilateral

132099.2   IX (Glossopharyngeal nerve) NFS
132002.2   contusion
132004.2   laceration

132299.2   X (Vagus nerve, excluding injury in neck or abdomen) NFS
132202.2   contusion
132204.2   laceration

132499.2   XI (Spinal accessory nerve) NFS
132402.2   contusion
132404.2   laceration

132699.2   XII (Hypoglossal nerve) NFS
132602.2   contusion
132604.2   laceration

コード	損傷内容

130699.2　Ⅱ（視神経－頭蓋内および視神経管内）　詳細不明

> 眼窩内の視神経損傷は顔面損傷としてコードを選択する。損傷部位が特定されていない場合は頭部損傷としてコードを選択する。

130602.2　　　　挫傷
130604.2　　　　　　両側
130606.2　　　　裂傷
130608.2　　　　　　両側

130899.2　Ⅲ（動眼神経）　詳細不明
130802.2　　　　挫傷または圧迫（テント切痕ヘルニアによる損傷を含む）
130804.2　　　　裂傷

131099.2　Ⅳ（滑車神経）　詳細不明
131002.2　　　　挫傷
131004.2　　　　裂傷

131299.2　Ⅴ（三叉神経）　詳細不明
131202.2　　　　挫傷
131204.2　　　　裂傷

131499.2　Ⅵ（外転神経）　詳細不明
131402.2　　　　挫傷
131404.2　　　　裂傷

131699.2　Ⅶ（顔面神経）　詳細不明
131602.2　　　　挫傷
131604.2　　　　裂傷

131899.2　Ⅷ（内耳神経，聴神経と前庭神経を含む）　詳細不明
131802.2　　　　挫傷
131804.2　　　　裂傷
131806.2　　　　　　両側

132099.2　Ⅸ（舌咽神経）　詳細不明
132002.2　　　　挫傷
132004.2　　　　裂傷

132299.2　Ⅹ（迷走神経，頸部および腹部での損傷を除く）　詳細不明
132202.2　　　　挫傷
132204.2　　　　裂傷

132499.2　Ⅺ（副神経）　詳細不明
132402.2　　　　挫傷
132404.2　　　　裂傷

132699.2　Ⅻ（舌下神経）　詳細不明
132602.2　　　　挫傷
132604.2　　　　裂傷

HEAD (cranium and brain)

CODE	INJURY DESCRIPTION

INTERNAL ORGANS

> The injuries in this section should be coded only if verified by CT scan, MRI, surgery, x-ray, angiography or autopsy. Clinical diagonosis alone is not an adequate determination for establishing the existence of an anatomic lesion for coding purposes.

140299.5	**Brain stem** (hypothalamus, medulla, midbrain, pons) NFS
140202.5	compression (includes transtentorial (uncal) or cerebellar tonsillar herniation)
140204.5	contusion
140206.5	diffuse axonal injury (white matter shearing)

> Use this code if (1) DAI is described as "white matter shearing" or (2) if the specific term "diffuse axonal injury" is ascribed by a physician to the brain injury. If neither (1) nor (2) is present, use the sections on "Length of Unconsciousness" or "Loss of Consciousness" to code prolonged LOC. LOC must be directly related to documented head injury.

140208.5	infarction
140210.5	injury involving hemorrhage
140212.6	laceration
140214.6	massive destruction (crush)
140216.6	penetrating injury
140218.6	transection
140499.3	**Cerebellum** NFS

> Use this section only if cerebellum, infratentorial or posterior fossa are named. Otherwise, code as Cerebrum.

140402.3	contusion, single or multiple, NFS [include perilesional edema for size]
140403.3	small (superficial; ≤15cc; ≤3cm diameter)
140404.4	large (15-30cc; >3cm diameter)
140405.5	extensive (massive; total volume >30cc)
140406.5	diffuse axonal injury

> Use this code if (1) DAI is described as "white matter shearing" or (2) if the specific term "diffuse axonal injury" is ascribed by a physician to the brain injury. If neither (1) nor (2) is present, use the sections on "Length of Unconsciousness" or "Loss of Consciousness" to code prolonged LOC. LOC must be directly related to documented head injury.

140410.4	hematoma (hemorrhage) NFS

> Use this code for "extra axial" unless further described as epidural or subdural.

140414.4	epidural or extradural NFS [include perilesional edema for size]
140418.4	small (≤30cc in adults;[a] ≤1cm thick[a]; smear; tiny; moderate)
140422.5	large (>30cc in adults;[b] >1cm thick[b]; massive; extensive)
140426.4	intracerebellar including petechial and subcortical NFS [include surrounding edema for size]
140430.4	small (≤15cc; ≤3cm diameter)
140434.5	large (>15cc; >3cm diameter)
140438.4	subdural NFS
140442.4	small (≤30cc in adults[a]; ≤1cm thick[a]; smear; tiny; moderate)
140446.5	large (>30cc in adults;[b] >1cm thick[b]; massive; extensive)

---

[a] ≤15cc or ≤2cm diameter/thick if ≤10 years old.
[b] >15cc or >2cm diameter/thick if ≤10 years old.

頭部（頭蓋と脳）

コード	損傷内容

脳

この章における損傷コードを選択するためには，損傷部位がCTスキャン，MRI，手術，X線，血管造影，剖検などによって裏付けられている必要がある。コード選択にさいして，臨床診断のみで解剖学的損傷部位を確定するのは適切ではない。

コード		損傷内容
140299.5	**脳幹**（視床下部，延髄，中脳，橋）	詳細不明
140202.5		圧迫（テント切痕〔鉤〕ヘルニア，小脳扁桃ヘルニアを含む）
140204.5		挫傷
140206.5		びまん性軸索損傷（白質剪断）

上のコードは，(1)"白質剪断"と記載されている場合，あるいは(2)臨床医が"びまん性軸索損傷（DAI）"を明確な定義のある用語として用いた場合に使用する。(1)でも(2)でもない場合，"意識消失の時間"の章，あるいは「意識レベル」の章のコードを選択する。「意識消失」は直接，頭部外傷によるものでなければならない。

140208.5	梗塞
140210.5	出血を伴う損傷
140212.6	裂傷
140214.6	広範囲損傷（挫滅）
140216.6	穿通性損傷
140218.6	離断

| 140499.3 | **小脳** 詳細不明 | 小脳，テント下，後頭蓋窩の損傷のみ以下のコードを選択する。その他は大脳の損傷としてコードを選択する。 |

140402.3	挫傷，単発または多発［周囲の浮腫を含めた大きさ］ 詳細不明
140403.3	小（表在性；出血量が15ml以下；直径3 cm以下）
140404.4	大（出血量15～30ml；直径が3 cmを超える）
140405.5	広範囲（大量；出血量が30mlを超える）

| 140406.5 | びまん性軸索損傷 |

上のコードは，(1)"白質剪断"と記載されている場合，あるいは(2)臨床医が"びまん性軸索損傷（DAI）"を明確な定義のある用語として用いた場合に使用する。(1)でも(2)でもない場合，"意識消失の時間"の章，あるいは「意識レベル」の章のコードを選択する。「意識消失」は直接，頭部外傷によるものでなければならない。

| 140410.4 | 血腫（出血） 詳細不明 |

上のコードは，脳実質外の血腫であるが，硬膜外血腫あるいは硬膜下血腫と特定できる根拠がない場合に使用する。

140414.4	硬膜外血腫［周囲の浮腫を含めた大きさ］ 詳細不明
140418.4	小（成人[a]では出血量が30ml以下；厚さ[a]が1 cm以下；薄い；少量；中程度）
140422.5	大（成人[b]では出血量が30mlを超える；厚さ[b]が1 cmを超える；大量；広範囲）

140426.4	点状出血および皮質下出血を含む小脳出血［周囲の浮腫を含めた大きさ］ 詳細不明
140430.4	小（出血量が15ml以下；直径が3 cm以下）
140434.5	大（出血量が15mlを超える；直径が3 cmを超える）

140438.4	硬膜下血腫 詳細不明
140442.4	小（成人[a]では出血量が30ml以下；厚さ[a]が1 cm以下；薄い；少量；中程度）
140446.5	大（成人[b]では出血量が30mlを超える；厚さ[b]が1 cmを超える；大量；広範囲）

---

[a] 10歳以下では出血量が15ml以下または血腫の大きさが直径または厚さ2 cm以下。
[b] 10歳以下では出血量が15mlを超えるかまたは血腫の大きさが直径または厚さ2 cmを超える。

HEAD (cranium and brain)

CODE	INJURY DESCRIPTION

Cerebellum (continued)

injury involving any of the following but not further specified anatomically other than cerebellum, infratentorial or posterior fossa:

> Use this category even in the presence of anatomically described injuries but only if substantiated.

140450.3   brain swelling/edema not including perilesional edema NFS (directly related to head trauma, not anoxia or other nontraumatic cause)

> Code one or other, i. e., swelling or edema, but not both.

140458.3   infarction (acute due to traumatic vascular occlusion)
140462.3   ischemia
140466.3   subarachnoid hemorrhage
140470.3   subpial hemorrhage

140474.4   laceration

140478.5   penetrating injury

140699.3   **Cerebrum** NFS   Use if described as "brain" injury

140602.3   contusion NFS [include pericontusional edema for size]
140604.3   single NFS
140606.3   small (superficial; ($\leq$30cc[a]; $\leq$4cm diameter[a]; midline shift $\leq$5mm)
140608.4   large (deep; 30-50cc[b]; >4cm diameter[b]; midline shift >5mm)

140610.5   extensive (massive; >50ccc)

140612.3   multiple, on same side but NFS
140614.3   small (superficial; total volume $\leq$30cc;[a] midline shift $\leq$5mm)
140616.4   large (total volume 30-50cc; midline shift >5mm)
140618.5   extensive (massive; total volume >50cc[c])

140611.3   multiple NFS

140620.3   multiple, at least one on each side but NFS
140622.3   small (superficial; total volume $\leq$30cc)
140624.4   large (total volume 30-50cc)
140626.5   extensive (massive; total volume >50cc)

140628.5   diffuse axonal injury

> Use this code if (1) DAI is described as "white matter shearing" or (2) if the specific term "diffuse asonal injury" is ascribed by a physician to the brain injury. If neither (1) nor (2) is present, use the sections on "Length of Unconsciousness" or "Loss of Consciousness" to code prolonged LOC. LOC must be directly related to documented head injury.

140629.4   hematoma (hemorrhage) NFS

> Use this code for "extra axial" unless further described as epidural or subdural.

---

[a] $\leq$15cc or $\leq$2cm diameter/thick if $\leq$10 years old.
[b] 15-30cc or 2-4cm diameter/thick if $\leq$10 years old.
[c] >30cc or >4cm diameter/thick if $\leq$10 years old.

コード	損傷内容

小脳（続き）

以下のコードは小脳，テント下または後頭蓋窩に損傷があるが，前記の損傷が特定できない場合にのみ選択する。

> ただしこれは解剖学的に損傷が確認されている場合にのみ使う。

140450.3 　　脳腫脹／浮腫　ただし損傷周囲の浮腫は含まない　詳細不明
　　　　　　　（酸素欠乏や他の外傷以外の原因による場合は使用しない）

> 上のコードはどちらか一方にだけ使用し，例えば腫脹または浮腫として，両方を併記しない。

140458.3 　　梗塞（外傷性血管閉塞による急性のもの）
140462.3 　　虚血
140466.3 　　くも膜下出血
140470.3 　　軟膜下出血

140474.4 　　裂傷

140478.5 　　穿通性損傷

140699.3 **大脳**　詳細不明　　"脳"の損傷と記載された場合に用いる。
140602.3 　　挫傷　[周囲の浮腫を含めた大きさ]　詳細不明
140604.3 　　　　単発性　詳細不明
140606.3 　　　　　　小（表在性；30ml 以下[a]；直径 4 cm 以下[a]；正中偏位が 5 mm 以下）
140608.4 　　　　　　大（深在性；30〜50ml[b]；直径 4 cm を超える[b]；正中偏位が 5 mm を超える）
140610.5 　　　　　　広範囲（大量；50ml[c] を超える）

140612.3 　　　　多発性（片側に存在）　詳細不明
140614.3 　　　　　　小（表在性；合計30ml 以下[a]；正中偏位が 5 mm 以下）
140616.4 　　　　　　大（合計30〜50ml；正中偏位が 5 mm を超える）
140618.5 　　　　　　広範囲（大量；合計50ml[c] を超える）

140611.3 　　　　多発性　詳細不明

140620.3 　　　　多発性（両側に存在）　詳細不明
140622.3 　　　　　　小（表在性；合計30ml 以下）
140624.4 　　　　　　大（合計30〜50ml）
140626.5 　　　　　　広範囲（大量；合計50ml を超える）

140628.5 　　びまん性軸索損傷

> 上のコードは，(1)"白質剪断"と記載されている場合，あるいは(2)臨床医が"びまん性軸索損傷（DAI）"を明確な定義のある用語として用いた場合に使用する。(1)でも(2)でもない場合，"意識消失の時間"の章，あるいは"意識レベル"の章のコードを選択する。「意識消失」は直接，頭部外傷によるものでなければならない。

140629.4 　　血腫（出血）　詳細不明

> 上のコードは，脳実質外の血腫であるが，硬膜外血腫あるいは硬膜下血腫と特定できる根拠がない場合に使用する。

---

[a] 10歳以下では出血量が15ml 以下または血腫の大きさが直径または厚さ 2 cm 以下。
[b] 10歳以下では出血量が15〜30ml または血腫の大きさが直径または厚さ 2 〜 4 cm。
[c] 10歳以下では出血量が30ml を超えるかまたは血腫の大きさが直径または厚さ 4 cm を超える。

HEAD (cranium and brain)

CODE	INJURY DESCRIPTION

Cerebrum (continued)

Code	Description
140630.4	epidural or extradural NFS (include perilesional hematoma for size)
140632.4	small (≤50cc adult; ≤25cc if ≤10 year old; ≤1cm thick; smear; tiny; moderate)
140634.5	bilateral
140636.5	large (>50cc adult; >25cc if ≤10 years old; >1cm thick; massive; extensive)
140638.4	intracerebral NFS (include surrounding edema for size)
140640.4	small (≤30cc; ≤4cm diameter[a])
140642.4	petechial hemorrhage (s)
140644.4	subcortical hemorrhage
140646.5	bilateral
140648.5	large (>30cc; >4cm diameter[b])
140650.4	subdural NFS
140652.4	small (≤50cc adult; ≤25cc if ≤10 years old; ≤1cm thick; smear; tiny; moderate)
140654.5	bilateral
140656.5	large (>50cc adult; >25cc if ≤10 years old; >1cm thick; massive; extensive)

injury involving any of the following but not further specified anatomically other than cerebrum, supratentorial, anterior cranial fossa or middle cranial fossa:

> Use this category even in the presence of anatomically described injuries, but only if substantiated.

Code	Description
140660.3	brain swelling/edema not including perilesional edema NFS (directly related to head trauma, not anoxia or other nontraumatic cause)

> Code one or other, i. e. brain swelling or edema, but not both.

Code	Description
140662.3	mild (compressed ventricle (s) w/o compressed brain stem cisterns)
140664.4	moderate (compressed ventricle (s) and brain stem cisterns)
140666.5	severe (absent ventricle (s) or brain stem cisterns)
140676.3	infarction (acute due to traumatic vascular occlusion)
140678.4	intraventricular hemorrhage/intracerebral hematoma in ventricular system
140680.3	ischemia (directly related to trauma)
140682.3	pneumocephalus (directly related to trauma)
140684.3	subarachnoid hemorrhage
140686.3	subpial hemorrhage
140688.4	laceration
140690.5	penetrating injury
140799.3	**Pituitary** injury

---

[a] ≤15cc or ≤2cm diameter/thick if ≤10 years old.
[b] >15cc or >2cm diameter/thick if ≤10 years old.

頭部（頭蓋と脳）

コード	損傷内容

大脳（続き）

140630.4	硬膜外（周囲の血腫も含めた大きさ）　詳細不明
140632.4	小（成人では出血量が50ml以下；10歳以下では25ml以下；厚さが1 cm以下；薄い；小さい；中程度）
140634.5	両側
140636.5	大（成人では出血量が50mlを超える；10歳以下では25mlを超える；厚さが1 cmを超える；多量；広範囲）
140638.4	脳内血腫（周囲の血腫も含めた大きさ）　詳細不明
140640.4	小（30ml以下；直径4 cm以下[a]）
140642.4	点状出血
140644.4	皮質下出血
140646.5	両側
140648.5	大（30mlを超える；直径4 cm[b]を超える）
140650.4	硬膜下　詳細不明
140652.4	小（成人では出血量が50ml以下；10歳以下では25ml以下；厚さが1 cm以下；薄い；小さい；中程度）
140654.5	両側
140656.5	大（成人では出血量が50mlを超える；10歳以下では25mlを超える；厚さが1 cmを超える；多量；広範囲）

以下のコードには大脳，テント上，前頭蓋窩または中頭蓋窩以外には損傷があるが，前記の損傷が特定できない場合にのみ選択する

> ただしこれは解剖学的に損傷が確認されている場合にのみ選択する。

| 140660.3 | 脳腫脹／浮腫　ただし損傷周囲の浮腫は含まない　詳細不明 （酸素欠乏や外傷以外の原因による場合は使用しない） |

> 上のコードはどちらか一方にだけ使用し，例えば腫脹または浮腫として，両方を併記しない。

140662.3	軽症（脳室の圧迫はあるが脳幹周囲槽の圧迫はない）
140664.4	中等症（脳室と脳幹周囲槽の圧迫）
140666.5	重症（脳室または脳幹周囲槽の消失）
140676.3	梗塞（外傷性血管閉塞による急性のもの）
140678.4	脳室内出血／脳室穿破を主とする脳内血腫
140680.3	虚血（外傷に直接関連する）
140682.3	気脳症（外傷に直接関連する）
140684.3	くも膜下出血
140686.3	軟膜下出血
140688.4	裂傷
140690.5	穿通性損傷
140799.3	**脳下垂体**損傷

---

[a] 10歳以下では出血量が15ml以下または血腫の大きさが直径または厚さ2 cm以下。
[b] 10歳以下では出血量が15mlを超えるかまたは血腫の大きさが直径または厚さ2 cmを超える。

HEAD (cranium and brain)

CODE	INJURY DESCRIPTION

SKELETAL

Code all skull fractures under vault unless specified as base. Code associated brain or cranial nerve injuries separately under Nerves, Vessels or Organs. Code naso-orbito-ethmoidal fracture as basilar. In these cases, do not code facial fractures separately.

150200.3 **Base** (basilar) fracture NFS (may involve ethmoid, orbital roof, sphenoid, temporal--including petrous, squamous or mastoid portions--or occipital bones)
150202.3   without CSF leak
150204.3   with CSF leak

150206.4   complex (open[d] with torn, exposed or loss of brain tissue; comminuted; ring; hinge)

Any of the following clinical signs of basilar skull fracture linked to a stated clinical diagonosis in the medical chart can be used to corroborate its presence: hemotympanum; perforated tympanic membrane with blood in canal; mastoid hematoma (battle signs) ; CSF otorrhea; rhinorrhea; periorbital ecchymosis (raccoon's eyes).

150400.2 **Vault** fracture NFS (may involve frontal, occipital, parietal, sphenoid, or temporal bones)
150402.2   closed; simple; undisplaced; diastatic; linear
150404.3   comminuted; compound[d] (i. e. open but dura intact) ; depressed ≤2cm; displaced

150406.4   complex; open[d] with torn, exposed or loss of brain tissue
150408.4   massively depressed (large areas of skull depressed >2cm)

---

[d] The term "compound" is uniquely applied to skull fracture. It means open fracture. "Open" skull fracture means compound fracture plus torn, exposed or loss of brain tissue.

コード	損傷内容

骨 格

頭蓋骨骨折は，頭蓋底骨折と記載されていない限り，頭蓋冠骨折としてコードを選択する。また，合併する脳損傷，脳神経損傷は神経，血管または器官として別個にコードを選択する。鼻腔－眼窩－篩骨骨折は頭蓋底骨折としてコードを選択する。この場合，顔面骨折として別個にコードを選択してはいけない。

150200.3 **頭蓋底**骨折（篩骨，眼窩上壁，蝶型骨，側頭骨（岩様骨，鱗部，乳様突起を含む），後頭骨を含む）　詳細不明
150202.3 　　　髄液漏を伴わない
150204.3 　　　髄液漏を伴う

150206.4 　　　複雑（脳組織の裂傷，露出あるいは脱出を伴う開放骨折[d]，粉砕骨折，環状骨折，蝶番骨折）

診療録に以下の臨床症状が記載されていれば，頭蓋底骨折の存在を強く疑う根拠となる：鼓室内出血；外耳道への出血を伴う鼓膜穿孔；乳様突起の血腫（battle signs）；髄液耳漏；髄液鼻漏；眼窩周囲の斑状出血（raccoon's eyes）。

150400.2 **頭蓋冠**骨折（前頭骨，後頭骨，頭頂骨，蝶形骨，側頭骨を含む）　詳細不明
150402.2 　　　閉鎖性；単純；偏位なし；縫合離解；線状
150404.3 　　　粉砕；compound[d]（骨折部が露出しているが硬膜損傷を伴わない）；2 cm 以下の陥没；偏位あり
150406.4 　　　複雑；脳組織の裂傷，露出あるいは脱出を伴う開放骨折[d]
150408.4 　　　広範囲陥没（大きな面積にわたって 2 cm を超える陥没）

---

[d] 頭蓋における開放骨折は一般の開放骨折とは別の意味で用いられ，脳組織の裂傷，露出あるいは脱出が加わった骨折のことである。一般の開放骨折に相当する皮膚に孔が開き骨折部が露出している場合は，頭蓋骨骨折に限り使用される「compound 骨折」という語を用いる。

HEAD (cranium and brain)

GUIDELINES ON WHEN TO USE LOSS OF CONSCIOUSNESS INFORMATION

Unconsciousness is synonymous with coma and is defined as the inability to follow commands and no eye opening to any stimulation and no word verbalizations (non-word utterances can occur, i. e., grunts, groans). Loss of consciousness cannot be coded until it is determined that the coma is directly related to a brain injury and has lasted for at least 24 hours. Therefore, loss of consciousness codes cannot be used if: (1) death occurs within 24 hours and patient has not regained consciousness or (2) a "closed head injury" description is given with no information about LOC or length of unconsciousness except for descriptors 160820.4, 160822.5 or 160824.5. In such cases of inadequate information, use 115099.9 or 115999.9. These designators allow a means for identifying the occurrence of a head injury although calculation of an accurate ISS is not possible.

The Glasgow Coma Score is included under the "Level of Consciousness" section only as one indicator of neurologic status that needs corroboration for the presence of brain injury. The presence of alcohol or other drugs will oftentimes confound the assessment of brain injury based upon neurologic status. Similarly, intubation of patients following injury limits the application of the GCS to assess the presence or absence of brain injury. For these reasons, the GCS should never be used as the sole indicator of brain injury based on level of consciousness. Furthermore, LOC cannot be used as a descriptor of brain injury until at least 24 hours post injury unless the patient awakens within 24 hours. After 24 hours the effects of alcohol will have disappeared so that the presence or absence of brain injury can be determined. Also after 24 hours, other diagnostic procedures will have substantiated brain injury to obviate the need to code brain injury based on LOC.

Anatomical lesions
For coding head injuries other than those to the skull, the coder may know the anatomical lesion, the level of consciousness, or the duration of unconsciousness. If an anatomical lesion is substantiated by autopsy, CT scan, MRI (magnetic resonance imaging), surgery, x-ray, or angiography, it should be coded using the section titled internal Organs. [Recall that clinical diagnosis alone is not an adequate determination for establishing the existence of an anatomical lesion for coding purposes.]

Where loss of consciousness (LOC) accompanies a documented anatomical lesion, the LOC should be considered only if it reflects a more serious injury than is described by the anatomical lesion alone. In these cases, the higher AIS should be assigned to the injury.

Non-anatomical injury
In the absence of a documented anatomic lesion, only information on status of consciousness may be available to the coder. In these cases, the following sections on length of unconsciousness or level of consciousness should be used.

Self-reported brief LOC or reports of bystanders with no corroboration by EMS or medical personnel and no evidence of head trauma should be disregarded. Abrasions, contusions or lacerations to the scalp are coded under Whole Area and are not automatically presumed to have an associated brain injury.

Neurological deficit
One or more of the following sequela that was not present pre-injury constitute a neurological deficit if it lasts for more than a transient period (i. e., minutes) : hemiparesis; hemiplegia; weakness; sensory loss; hypesthesia; visual field defect; aphasia; dysphasia; seizure; central (not peripheral) facial weakness or palsy; deviation of both eyes to the same side; unequal pupils; pupils fixed or not reactive. The latter three must be due to head, not eye or orbital, injury.

LENGTH OF UNCONSCIOUSNESS

This section may be used only within the immediately preceding guidelines. This section should always be used in preference to the one that follows, called Level of Consciousness. The necessity to use this section in preference to the one titled Internal Organs (pages 5-7) oftentimes reflects inadequate date sources.

CODE	INJURY DESCRIPTION
	Unconsciousness known to be
160202.2	<1 hr.
160204.3	with neurological deficit
160206.3	1-6 hrs. unconsciousness
160208.4	with neurological deficit
160210.4	6-24 hrs. unconsciousness (includes 1 calendar day when hours cannot be estimated)
160212.5	with neurological deficit
160214.5	>24 hrs. unconsciousness

頭部（頭蓋と脳）

意識消失の情報に関するガイドライン

　意識消失とは昏睡と同じ意味であり，指示に対し従わず，かつ，どのような刺激にも開眼せず，かつ，単語の発語がない（言葉にならない発音はあってもよい，例えば，呻き声，唸り声など）状態と定義される。昏睡が直接脳損傷に関係したものであって，少なくとも24時間は持続していることが確定するまでは，意識消失のコードは用いることができない。したがって次の場合，意識消失のコードは選択できない。(1)24時間以内に意識が回復することなく死亡した患者。(2)160820.4，160822.5，160824.5のコードを例外として，意識障害や意識消失の長さについて何の情報もなく「閉鎖性頭部損傷」とだけ記載されている患者。そのような不十分な情報しかない場合は115099.9あるいは115999.9を用いる。これらのコードによって，正確なISSを計算することはできないが，脳損傷の存在を認識することはできる。

　Glasgow Coma Score（GCS）は「意識レベル」の章で用いられるが，神経学的状態の一指標とするためには脳損傷が存在するという確証を必要とする。アルコールや他の薬物の存在は神経学的状態に基づいた脳損傷の診断をしばしば混乱させる。同様に，外傷患者に気管挿管をすることによって，GCSを用いることに制限ができてしまい，脳損傷の有無を判断できなくなってしまう。このような理由から，GCSを単独の指標として用いて，意識レベルに基づいた脳損傷の評価を行ってはならない。さらに，患者が24時間以内に覚醒しない場合は，損傷後少なくとも24時間を経過するまでは，意識障害は脳損傷のコードとしては使用できない。アルコールの影響が消える24時間後脳損傷の有無が判断できるようになる。また24時間後には，他の診断手技に基づいてコード選択が可能になり，あえて意識障害に基づいて選択する必要がなくなるかもしれない。
　（訳注：ここでのGCSは，Glasgow Come Scale 合計点の意味で用いられている）

解剖学的に損傷部位が認められる場合
　頭蓋骨損傷以外の頭部外傷では，コード選択者は解剖学的な損傷部位，意識レベル，あるいは意識消失時間などの情報をもとにコードを選択することになる。もし解剖学的な損傷部位がCTスキャン，MRI，手術，X線撮影または血管造影によって確認できるならば，その解剖学上の各器官に選択されたコードを優先する［言い換えるとコードを選択することを目的にして臨床診断のみから解剖学的な損傷部位を決めることは適当でない］。

　解剖学的に損傷部位が確認できても，それに比べて意識消失（LOC）がより重症の場合には，本章のコードを選択する。

解剖学的に損傷部位が認められない場合
　解剖学的な損傷の確認ができない場合は，コード選択者にとって意識の状態に関する情報しか利用できない。そのような場合には「意識消失の時間」あるいは「意識レベル」の章に従う。

　自己申告による短時間の意識消失や，救急隊員，医療従事者による証明がなく，頭部外傷の証拠もない場合の目撃者の話は無視すべきである。そのさい「全域」にある頭皮の擦過傷，挫傷または裂創のコードを選択しても，自動的に脳損傷を伴うと思いこんではいけない。

神経脱落症状
　受傷前には認められなかった以下のような症状が，数分以上にわたり断続的あるいはそれ以上続く場合は，神経学的な障害が存在する：不全片麻痺；片麻痺；脱力；知覚麻痺；知覚鈍麻；視野狭窄；失語症；嚥下困難；けいれん発作；中枢性（末梢性は除く）顔面脱力または麻痺；共同偏視；瞳孔不同；瞳孔固定または対光反射消失。最後の3項目は眼球または眼窩の損傷によるものではなく脳損傷によるものでなければならない。

意識消失の時間

この章は上述のガイドラインに沿ってのみ使用する。しかも後述する「意識レベル」をより優先しなければならない。「脳」の章よりこの章を優先して使用するとしばしば不正確なデータとなる。

コード	損傷内容
	意識消失の時間が次のとおり
160202.2	1時間未満
160204.3	神経脱落症状を伴う
160206.3	1～6時間
160208.4	神経脱落症状を伴う
160210.4	6～24時間（時間単位の推測が困難なときは，1日を含む）
160212.5	神経脱落症状を伴う
160214.5	24時間を超える

HEAD (cranium and brain)

LEVEL OF CONSCIOUSNESS

This section is used only if an injury cannot be coded by the Internal Organs (pages 5-7) or Length of Unconsciousness (page 9) sections. This level of consciousness and its duration must be observed by emergency or medical personnel, and must be related to head injury. The necessity to use this section in preference to the one titled Internal Organs oftentimes reflects inadequate date sources.

CODE	INJURY DESCRIPTION
160499.1	**Awake post resuscitation or on Initial Observation at Scene** (GCS[e] 15) NFS
160402.1	no prior unconsciousness, but may have headache or dizziness known to be a result of head injury
160404.2	with neurological deficit
160406.2	prior unconsciousness, but length of time NFS
160408.3	with neurological deficit
160410.2	amnesia (no recollection of injury)
160412.3	with neurological deficit
160414.2	unconsciousness known to be <1 hr.
160416.3	with neurological deficit
160699.2	**Lethargic, Stuporous, Obtunded post resuscitation or on Initial Observation at Scene** (Can Be Aroused by Verbal or Painful Stimuli; GCS[e] 9-14) NFS
160602.2	no prior unconsciousness
160604.3	with neurological deficit
160606.2	prior unconsciousness but length of time NFS
160608.3	with neurological deficit
160610.2	unconsciousness known to be <1 hr.
160612.3	with neurological deficit
160614.3	1-6 hrs. unconsciousness
160616.4	with neurological deficit
160899.3	**Unconscious post resuscitation or on Initial Observation at Scene** (Unresponsive to Verbal Command or Painful Stimuli; GCS[e] ≤8) NFS
160802.2	length of unconsciousness NFS
160804.3	with neurological deficit
	unconsciousness known to be
160806.3	<1 hr.
160808.4	with neurological deficit
160810.3	1-6 hrs. unconsciousness
160812.4	with neurological deficit
160814.4	6-24 hrs. unconsciousness (includes 1 calendar day when hours cannot be estimated)
160816.5	with neurological deficit
160818.5	>24 hrs. unconsciousness
160820.4	appropriate movements, but only upon painful stimuli no matter the length of unconsciousness
160822.5	with neurological deficit
160824.5	Inappropriate movements (decerebrate, decorticate, flaccid, no response to pain) no matter the length of unconsciousness

CONCUSSION

161000.2 **Cerebral concussion**

> Use only in those cases where there is convincing evidence of head injury and where the medical diagnosis is made by a physician and is given simply as "concussion" with no other description or clarification.

---

[e] Glasgow Coma Score in the absence of hypotension.

頭部（頭蓋と脳）

意識レベル

前述の「脳」（28〜30ページ）または「意識消失の時間」（32ページ）によってコードを選択することが不可能な場合にのみ本章のコードを選択する。意識レベルとその期間は救急隊員または医療関係者によって観察される必要があり，頭部外傷に基づくものでなければならない。「脳」の章より本章を優先して使用するとしばしば不正確なデータとなる。

コード	損傷内容
160499.1	救急蘇生後または初診時に覚醒状態である（GCS[e] 15）　詳細不明
160402.1	初診以前に意識消失はなかったが，頭部外傷による頭痛，眩暈がある
160404.2	神経脱落症状を伴う
160406.2	初診以前に意識消失はあったが，その期間が不明
160408.3	神経脱落症状を伴う
160410.2	健忘症（受傷状況を覚えていない）
160412.3	神経脱落症状を伴う
160414.2	1時間未満の意識消失
160416.3	神経脱落症状を伴う
160699.2	救急蘇生後または現場での最初の観察時に嗜眠，昏迷，鈍麻である（言葉または痛み刺激によって覚醒する：GCS[e] 9〜14）　詳細不明
160602.2	初診以前に意識消失はなかった
160604.3	神経脱落症状を伴う
160606.2	初診以前に意識消失はあったが，その期間が不明
160608.3	神経脱落症状を伴う
160610.2	1時間未満の意識消失
160612.3	神経脱落症状を伴う
160614.3	1〜6時間の意識消失
160616.4	神経脱落症状を伴う
160899.3	救急蘇生後または現場での最初の観察時に意識消失である（言葉による指示，または痛み刺激に対する反応なし：GCS[e] 8以下）　詳細不明
160802.2	意識消失の時間　詳細不明
160804.3	神経脱落症状を伴う
	意識消失が次の通り
160806.3	1時間未満
160808.4	神経脱落症状を伴う
160810.3	1〜6時間の意識消失
160812.4	神経脱落症状を伴う
160814.4	6〜24時間の意識消失（時間単位の推測が困難なときは，1日を含む）
160816.5	神経脱落症状を伴う
160818.5	24時間を超える意識消失
160820.4	痛み刺激に対してのみ適切な動作がある。意識消失の時間は問わない
160822.5	神経脱落症状を伴う
160824.5	不適切な動作（除脳硬直，除皮質硬直，全身弛緩状態，痛み刺激に対する反応なし）意識消失の時間は問わない

脳震盪

161000.2	脳震盪

頭部外傷であることについて説得力のある証拠があり，医師により医学的診断が単純に"脳震盪"だけで，他に記載や説明がない場合にのみ使用する。

---

[e] 低血圧症を認めていない状態でのGCSを示す。

顔　面
（耳と目を含む）

FACE (includes ear and eye)

CODE	INJURY DESCRIPTION

WHOLE AREA

216000.1	**Penetrating injury** NFS
216002.1	superficial; minor
216004.2	with tissue loss $>25cm^2$
216006.3	with blood loss $>20\%$ by volume

If deeper structures are involved, code under Vessels, Organs or Skeletal.

Assign one of the following codes, as appropriate, to soft tissue (external) injuries to the face. To calculate an ISS, however, assign these injuries to the External body region and follow rules for ISS calculation on pages xviii and xix.

210099.1	**Skin/Subcutaneous/muscle** (including eyelid, lip, external ear, forehead) NFS
210202.1	abrasion
210402.1	contusion
210600.1	laceration NFS
210602.1	minor; superficial
210604.2	major ($>10cm$ long and into subcutaneous tissue)
210606.3	blood loss $>20\%$ by volume
210800.1	avulsion NFS
210802.1	superficial; minor ($\leq 25cm^2$)
210804.2	major ($>25cm^2$ but blood loss $\leq 20\%$ by volume)
210806.3	blood loss $>20\%$ by volume

Use one of the following two descriptors when such vague information is the only information available. These descriptors allow a means for identifying the occurrence of face injury, but they do not allow the calculation of an accurate ISS in these patients.

215099.9	**Blunt/traumatic face** injury NFS
215999.9	Died without further evaluation; no autopsy

VESSELS   also see NECK

220200.1	**External carotid artery** branch(es) including facial and internal maxillary laceration NFS
220202.1	minor
220204.3	major (blood loss $>20\%$ by volume)

NERVES   also see CRANIAL NERVES under HEAD

230299.1	**Optic nerve** NFS intraorbital portion only; for intracranial portion or location unknown, code under cranial nerves in Head section
230202.2	contusion
230204.2	laceration
230206.2	avulsion

顔面（耳と目を含む）

コード	損傷内容

全　域

216000.1	**穿通性損傷**　詳細不明	
216002.1		表在性；小
216004.2		組織欠損が25cm²を超える
216006.3		出血量が全血液量の20％を超える

> もしも深部組織の損傷を伴う場合は，血管，内臓あるいは骨格のコードを選択する。

> 顔面の軟部組織（体表）の損傷には，以下のコードの中で適切なものを選択する。ただしISSを算出する場合には「体表」の区分として取り扱い，21，22ページのISS計算ルールに従う。

210099.1	**皮膚/皮下組織/筋肉**（眼瞼，口唇，外耳，前額部を含む）　詳細不明	
210202.1		擦過傷
210402.1		挫傷
210600.1		裂創　詳細不明
210602.1		小；表在性
210604.2		大（長さが10cmを超え，かつ皮下組織に達する）
210606.3		出血量が全血液量の20％を超える
210800.1		剥離　詳細不明
210802.1		表在性；小（25cm²以下）
210804.2		大（25cm²を超え，出血量が全血液量の20％以下）
210806.3		出血量が全血液量の20％を超える

> 不確定な情報しか得られない場合には，以下の2つのコードのうちいずれかを選択する。ただしこれらのコードを選択した場合にISSは計算してはならない。

215099.9	**鈍的顔面**損傷　詳細不明	
215999.9		死亡（詳細な評価なし）；剖検なし

血　管

> 頸部も参照

220200.1	**外頸動脈**の分枝の裂傷・裂創（顎動脈，顔面動脈含む）　詳細不明	
220202.1		小
220204.3		大（血液量の20％を超える）

神　経

> 頭部の脳神経の章も参照

230299.1	**視神経**　詳細不明	眼窩内の損傷に限る；頭蓋内もしくは，損傷の局在が不明の場合は頭部の脳神経のコードを選択する。
230202.2		挫傷
230204.2		裂傷
230206.2		断裂

FACE (includes ear and eye)

CODE	INJURY DESCRIPTION

INTERNAL ORGANS

240299.1	**Ear** NFS	
240204.1		Ear canal injury
240208.1		Inner or middle ear injury
240212.1		Ossicular chain (ear bone) dislocation
240216.1		Tympanic membrane (eardrum) rupture
240220.1		Vestibular apparatus injury
240499.1	**Eye** NFS	
240402.2		Eye avulsion (enucleation)
240408.1		Canaliculus (tear duct) laceration
240412.1		Choroid rupture
240416.1		Conjunctiva injury
240699.1		Cornea NFS
240602.1		abrasion
240604.1		contusion (includes hyphema)
240606.1		laceration
240800.1		Iris laceration
241000.1		Retina laceration (includes retinal hemorrhage with known injury to eye)
241002.2		with retinal detachment
241200.1		Sclera laceration
241202.2		involving globe (includes rupture)
241499.1		Uvea injury
241699.1		Vitreous injury
243099.1	**Mouth** NFS	
243299.1	**Gingiva** (gum) NFS	
243202.1		contusion
243204.1		laceration
243206.1		avulsion
243400.1	**Tongue** laceration NFS	
243402.1		superficial
243404.2		deep/extensive

SKELETAL

250200.2   **Alveolar ridge** (bone) fracture with or without injury to teeth
              Do not code teeth separately where these occur simultaneously
250400.1   **Facial bone** (s) fracture NFS

顔面（耳と目を含む）

コード	損傷内容

内　臓

240299.1	耳	詳細不明
240204.1		外耳道損傷
240208.1		内耳，中耳損傷
240212.1		耳小骨脱臼
240216.1		鼓膜破裂
240220.1		前庭器官損傷
240499.1	目	詳細不明
240402.2		眼球脱出（摘出）
240408.1		涙管裂傷・裂創
240412.1		脈絡膜破裂
240416.1		結膜損傷
240699.1		角膜　詳細不明
240602.1		擦過傷
240604.1		挫傷（前房出血含む）
240606.1		裂傷・裂創
240800.1		虹彩裂傷・裂創
241000.1		網膜裂傷・裂創（眼外傷に伴う網膜出血を含む）
241002.2		網膜剥離を伴う
241200.1		強膜裂傷・裂創
241202.2		眼球内に達する（眼球破裂を含む）
241499.1		ぶどう膜損傷
241699.1		硝子体損傷
243099.1	口	詳細不明
243299.1	歯肉	詳細不明
243202.1		挫傷
243204.1		裂傷・裂創
243206.1		剥離
243400.1	舌裂創	詳細不明
243402.1		表在性
243404.2		深在性／広範囲

骨　格

250200.2	**歯槽骨**骨折，歯牙損傷の有無を問わない
	ただし，同時に生じた場合は，歯牙損傷のコードは選択しない。
250400.1	**顔面骨**骨折　詳細不明

FACE (includes ear and eye)

CODE	INJURY DESCRIPTION

250699.1 **Mandible NFS** bilateral coded as single injury
                      dislocation code under Temporomandibular joint

250600.1   fracture NFS
250602.1   closed but NFS as to location
250604.1   body with or without ramus involvement
250606.1   ramus
250608.2   subcondylar
250610.2   open/displaced/comminuted any or combination but NFS as to location
250612.2   body with or without ramus involvement
250614.2   ramus
250616.2   subcondylar

250800.2 **Maxilla** fracture, any (including maxillary sinus) except Le Fort fractures as described below
                  bilateral coded as single injury
250804.2   Le Fort I [f]
250806.2   Le Fort II [g]
250808.3   Le Fort III [h]
250810.4   blood loss >20% by volume

251099.1 **Nose** NFS
251000.1   fracture NFS
251002.1   closed
251004.2   open/displaced/comminuted any or combination
251090.1   rupture of mucosa/vessels ("nosebleed", epitaxis)

251200.2 **Orbit** fracture NFS
251202.2   closed
251204.3   open/displaced/comminuted any or combination

251499.1 **Teeth** any number but NFS see also Alveolar ridge
251402.1   dislocation or loosened
251404.1   fracture
251406.1   avulsion

251699.1 **Temporomandibular joint** NFS
251602.1   sprain
251604.2   dislocation

251800.2 **Zygoma** fracture

---

[f] Le Fort I -horizontal segmented fracture of the alveolar process of the maxilla in which the teeth are usually contained in the detached portion of the bone.

[g] Le Fort II -unilateral or bilateral fracture of the maxilla in which the body of the maxilla is separated from the facial skeleton and the separated portion is pyramidal in shape; the fracture may extend through the body of the maxilla down the midline of the hard palate, through the floor of the orbit and into the nasal cavity.

[h] Le Fort III -a fracture in which the entire maxilla and one or more facial bones are completely separated from the base of the skull.

顔面（耳と目を含む）

コード	損傷内容

250699.1　**下顎骨**　詳細不明　両側性でも，１つの損傷としてコードを選択する。
　　　　　　　　　脱臼　顎関節のコードを選択する。

250600.1　　　　骨折　詳細不明
250602.1　　　　　　非開放，位置に関しては不明
250604.1　　　　　　　　下顎体部骨折（ただし下顎枝の骨折は問わない）
250606.1　　　　　　　　下顎枝
250608.2　　　　　　　　頸部
250610.2　　　　　　開放／転位／粉砕　いずれか１つ以上　位置に関しては不明
250612.2　　　　　　　　下顎体部骨折（ただし下顎枝の骨折は問わない）
250614.2　　　　　　　　下顎枝
250616.2　　　　　　　　頸部

250800.2　**上顎骨**骨折，以下記載の Le Fort 骨折を除くすべて（上顎洞を含む）
　　　　　　両側性でも，１つの損傷としてコードを選択する。
250804.2　　　　Le Fort Ⅰ型 [f]
250806.2　　　　Le Fort Ⅱ型 [g]
250808.3　　　　Le Fort Ⅲ型 [h]
250810.4　　　　出血量が全血液量の20%を超える。

251099.1　**鼻**　詳細不明
251000.1　　　　骨折　詳細不明
251002.1　　　　　　非開放
251004.2　　　　　　開放／転位／粉砕　いずれか１つ以上
251090.1　　　　粘膜／血管の破裂（"鼻血"，鼻出血）

251200.2　**眼窩**骨折　詳細不明
251202.2　　　　　　非開放
251204.3　　　　　　開放／転位／粉砕　いずれか１つ以上

251499.1　**歯牙**　（本数は問わない）　詳細不明　歯槽骨の項も参照
251402.1　　　　脱臼または動揺
251404.1　　　　破折
251406.1　　　　脱落

251699.1　**顎関節**　詳細不明
251602.1　　　　捻挫
251604.2　　　　脱臼

251800.2　**頬骨**骨折

---

[f] Le Fort Ⅰ型：上顎骨歯槽突起を水平方向に横切る骨折。通常，分離された骨片部分に歯牙が含まれている。

[g] Le Fort Ⅱ型：上顎骨が片側または両側性（左右）に骨折し，上顎骨体部は顔面骨格より遊離し，ピラミッド型を呈する。骨折は上顎骨体部を経て，硬口蓋正中に達し，上方は眼窩底より鼻腔に至る。

[h] Le Fort Ⅲ型：上顎骨全体および１つ以上の顔面骨が頭蓋底より完全に分離した骨折。

頸 部

NECK

CODE	INJURY DESCRIPTION

WHOLE AREA

311000.6 **Decapitation**

316000.1 **Penetrating injury** NFS
316002.1   superficial; minor
316004.2   with tissue loss $>100cm^2$ but blood loss $\leq 20\%$ by volume
316006.3   with blood loss $>20\%$ by volume

> If deeper structures are involved, code under Vessels, Internal Organs or Skeletal.

> Assign one of the following codes, as appropriate, to soft tissue (external) injuries to the neck. To calculate an ISS, however, assign these injuries to the External body region and follow rules for ISS calculation on pages xviii and xix.

310099.1 **Skin/Subcutaneous tissue/muscle** NFS
310202.1   abrasion
310402.1   contusion (hematoma)
310600.1   laceration NFS
310602.1   minor; superficial
310604.2   major ($>20cm$ long and into subcutaneous tissue)
310606.3   blood loss $>20\%$ by volume
310800.1   avulsion NFS
310802.1   minor; superficial ($\leq 100cm^2$)
310804.2   major ($>100cm^2$ but blood loss $<20\%$ by volume)
310806.3   blood loss $>20\%$ by volume

> Use one of the following two codes when such vague information is the only description available. These descriptors allow a means for identifying the occurrence of neck injury, but they do not although the calculation of an accurate ISS in these patients.

315099.9 **Blunt/traumatic neck injury** NFS
315999.9   Died without further evaluation; no autopsy

VESSELS

> Vessel injuries are coded as separate injuries if: (1) they are isolated injuries (i. e., no accompanying documented organ injury) or (2) accompanying organ injury does not include any vessel injury description or (3) named vessel injury occurs with organ injury and is higher in severity than descriptor for organ injury.
>
> The terms "laceration", "puncture" and "perforation" are oftentimes used interchangeably to describe vessel injuries. When "perforation" or "puncture" is used, code as laceration. Descriptions for vessel lacerations distinguish between complete and incomplete transection. See footnotes "i" and "j". Thrombosis includes any injury to the vessel resulting in its occlusion (e. g., intimal tear, dissection).

頸 部

コード	損傷内容

全 域

311000.6　断頭

316000.1　**穿通性損傷**　詳細不明
316002.1　　　　表在性；小さい
316004.2　　　　組織欠損が100cm^{2}を超えるが，出血量が全血液量の20％以下
316006.3　　　　出血量が全血液量の20％を超える

> もしも深部組織の損傷を伴う場合は，血管，内臓あるいは骨格のコードを選択する。

> 頸部の軟部組織（皮膚）の損傷には，以下のコードの中で適切なものを選択する。ただしISSを算出する場合には，「体表」の区分として取り扱い，21，22ページのISS計算ルールに従う。

310099.1　**皮膚／皮下組織／筋肉**　詳細不明
310202.1　　　　擦過傷
310402.1　　　　挫傷（血腫）
310600.1　　　　裂創　詳細不明
310602.1　　　　　小；表在性
310604.2　　　　　大（長さが20cmを超え，かつ皮下組織に達する）
310606.3　　　　　出血量が全血液量の20％を超える
310800.1　　　　剥離　詳細不明
310802.1　　　　　小；表在性（100cm^{2}以下）
310804.2　　　　　大（100cm^{2}を超えるが，出血量が全血液量の20％以下）
310806.3　　　　　出血量が全血液量の20％を超える

> 不確定な情報しか得られない場合には，以下の2つのコードのうちいずれかを選択する。ただしこれらのコードを選択した場合にISSは計算してはならない。

315099.9　**鈍的頸部損傷**　詳細不明
315999.9　　　　死亡（詳細な評価なし）；剖検なし

血 管

> 血管損傷は，以下の場合には独立した損傷としてコードを選択する。
> (1)単独血管損傷（臓器損傷がない血管損傷）
> (2)臓器損傷に血管損傷に関する記載がないとき
> (3)血管損傷と臓器損傷が合併していて，血管損傷の重症度が臓器損傷の重症度より高いとき
> 血管損傷を表わす場合，"裂傷""穿刺""穿孔"などの用語はしばしば同じような意味で用いられる。血管の"穿孔"や"穿刺"と記載されている場合は"裂傷"としてコード選択する。血管の裂傷については，完全断裂と不完全断裂に区分する。脚注 i，j を参照。血栓は閉塞（例；動脈内膜の裂傷，解離）となるすべての血管損傷も含む。

NECK

CODE	INJURY DESCRIPTION

NERVES

Brachial plexus see SPINE

Cervical spinal cord or nerve root see SPINE

330299.2   **Phrenic** injury

330499.1   **Vagus** injury also see THORAX and ABDOMEN

INTERNAL ORGANS

Esophagus see THORAX

340299.2   **Larynx**, including thyroid and cricoid cartilage, NFS
340202.2   contusion (hematoma)
340204.2   laceration, puncture NFS
340206.2   no perforation; partial thickness; mucosal tear
340208.3   perforation; full thickness but not complete transection
340210.4   with vocal cord involvement
340212.5   avulsion; crush; rupture; transection; massive destruction

340699.3   **Pharynx or Retropharyngeal area** NFS
340602.3   contusion (hematoma)
340604.2   laceration, puncture NFS
340606.3   no perforation; partial thickness; mucosal tear
340608.4   perforation; full thickness but not complete transection
340610.5   avulsion; crush; rupture; transection; massive destruction

341099.2   **Salivary gland** NFS
341002.3   with ductal involvement or transection

341499.1   **Thyroid gland** NFS
341402.1   contusion (hematoma)
341404.2   laceration

Trachea see THORAX

341899.2   **Vocal cord** NFS (not due to intubation)
341802.2   unilateral
341804.3   bilateral

SKELETAL

Cervical spine see SPINE

350200.2   **Hyoid** fracture

コード	損傷内容

神経

　　　　腕神経叢　　脊椎を参照

　　　　頸髄または神経根　　脊椎を参照

330299.2　横隔神経損傷

330499.1　迷走神経損傷　　胸部および腹部も参照

内臓

　　　　食道　　胸部を参照

340299.2　喉頭，甲状軟骨，輪状軟骨を含む　詳細不明
340202.2　　　挫傷（血腫）
340204.2　　　裂傷・裂創，穿刺　詳細不明
340206.2　　　　　穿孔なし；非全層性；粘膜裂傷
340208.3　　　　　穿孔あり；全層性，ただし完全断裂には至らない
340210.4　　　　　　声帯損傷を合併
340212.5　　　断裂；挫滅；破裂；離断；広範囲損傷

340699.3　咽頭または咽頭後部　詳細不明
340602.3　　　挫傷（血腫）
340604.2　　　裂傷・裂創，穿刺　詳細不明
340606.3　　　　　穿孔なし；非全層性；粘膜裂傷
340608.4　　　　　穿孔あり；全層性，ただし完全断裂には至らない
340610.5　　　断裂；挫滅；破裂；離断；広範囲損傷

341099.2　唾液腺　詳細不明
341002.3　　　導管の損傷，離断を伴う

341499.1　甲状腺　詳細不明
341402.1　　　挫傷（血腫）
341404.2　　　裂傷・裂創

　　　　気管　　胸部を参照

341899.2　声帯（気管挿管が原因でない）詳細不明
341802.2　　　片側
341804.3　　　両側

骨格

　　　　頸椎　　脊椎を参照

350200.2　舌骨骨折

胸　部

THORAX

CODE	INJURY DESCRIPTION

WHOLE AREA

411000.2   **Breast** avulsion, female

413000.6   Bilateral destruction of skeletal, vascular, organ and tissue systems ("crush" injury)

415000.4   **Open ("sucking") chest wound** (OIS Grade IV)

416000.1   **Penetrating injury** NFS
416002.1   superficial; minor; into pleural cavity but not involving deeper structures
416004.2   with tissue loss >100cm^2 but blood loss ≤20% by volume (OIS Grade III)
416006.3   with blood loss >20% by volume
416008.3   with hemo-/pneumothorax except tension PTX [see442210.5]

> If deeper structures are involved, code under Vessels, Internal Organs or Skeletal.

> Assign one of the following codes, as appropriate, to soft tissue (external) injuries to the thorax. To calculate an ISS, however, assign injuries in this category to the External body region and follow rules for ISS calclation on pages xviii and xix.

410099.1   **Skin/Subcutaneous/muscle/chest wall** NFS
410202.1   abrasion
410402.1   contusion (hematoma) (OIS Grade I)
410600.1   laceration NFS
410602.1   minor; superficial (OIS Grade I, II)
410604.2   major (>20cm long and into subcutaneous tissue)
410606.3   blood loss >20% by volume
410800.1   avulsion NFS
410802.1   minor; superficial; (≤100cm^2)
410804.2   major (>100cm^2 but blood loss <20% by volume)
410806.3   blood loss >20% by volume

> Use one of the following two descriptors when such vague information is the only descriptor available. These descriptors allow a means for identifying the occurrence of thoracic injury, but they do not allow the calculation of an accurate ISS in these patients.

415099.9   **Blunt/traumatic chest (thoracic) injury** NFS
415999.9   Died without further evaluation; no autopsy

VESSELS

> Vessel injuries are coded as separate injuries if: (1) they are isolated injuries (i. e., no accompanying documented organ injury) or (2) accompanying organ injury does not include any vessel injury description or (3) named vessel injury occurs with organ injury and is higher in severity than descriptor for organ injury.
> The terms "laceration", "puncture" and "perforation" are oftentimes used interchangeably to describe vessel injuries. When "perforation" or "puncture" is used, code as laceration. Descriptions for several vessel lacerations distinguish between complete and incomplete transection. See footnotes "i" and "j".

胸　部

コード	損傷内容

全　域

411000.2　**乳房**の剥離（女性）

413000.6　骨格，血管，臓器，組織系すべての両側性高度損傷（"挫滅"損傷）

415000.4　**開放性胸壁損傷**（吸い込み創）（OIS Grade Ⅳ）

416000.1　**穿通性損傷**　詳細不明
416002.1　　　　表在性；小；胸膜腔に達するが深部組織の損傷はない
416004.2　　　　組織欠損は100cm^{2}を超えるが，出血量が全血液量の20％以下（OIS Grade Ⅲ）
416006.3　　　　出血量が全血液量の20％を超える
416008.3　　　　血胸／気胸を伴う（緊張性気胸［442210.5参照］を除く）

> もしも深部組織の損傷を伴う場合は，血管，内臓あるいは骨格のコードを選択する。

> 胸部の軟部組織（体表）損傷には，以下のコードの中で適切なものを選択する。ただしISSを算出する場合には「体表」の区分として取り扱い，21，22ページのISS計算ルールに従う。

410099.1　**皮膚／皮下組織／筋肉／胸壁**　詳細不明
410202.1　　　　擦過傷
410402.1　　　　挫傷（血腫）（OIS Grade Ⅰ）
410600.1　　　　裂創　詳細不明
410602.1　　　　　　小；表在性（OIS Grade Ⅰ，Ⅱ）
410604.2　　　　　　大（長さが20cmを超え，かつ皮下組織に達する）
410606.3　　　　　　出血量が全血液量の20％を超える
410800.1　　　　剥離　詳細不明
410802.1　　　　　　小；表在性；（100cm^{2}以下）
410804.2　　　　　　大（100cm^{2}を超えるが，出血量が全血液量の20％を超えない）
410806.3　　　　　　出血量が全血液量の20％を超える

> 不確定な情報しか得られない場合には，以下の2つのコードのうちいずれかを選択する。ただしこれらのコードを選択した場合にISSは計算してはならない。

415099.9　**鈍的胸部損傷**　詳細不明
415999.9　　　　死亡（詳細な評価なし）；剖検なし

血　管

> 血管損傷は，以下の場合には独立した損傷としてコードを選択する。
> 　(1)単独血管損傷（臓器損傷がない血管損傷）
> 　(2)臓器損傷に血管損傷に関する記載がないとき
> 　(3)血管損傷と臓器損傷が合併していて，血管損傷の重症度が臓器損傷の重症度より高いとき
> 血管損傷を表わす場合，"裂傷""穿刺""穿孔"などの用語はしばしば同じような意味で用いられる。血管の"穿孔"や"穿刺"と記載されている場合は"裂傷"としてコード選択する。血管の裂傷については，完全断裂と不完全断裂に区分する。脚注 i，j を参照。

THORAX

CODE	INJURY DESCRIPTION
420299.4	**Aorta, thoracic,** NFS
420202.4	intimal tear, no disruption
420204.5	with aortic valve involvement
420206.4	laceration (perforation, puncture) NFS
420208.4	minor[i]
420210.5	major[j]
420212.5	with aortic root or valve involvement
420216.5	with hemorrhage confined to mediastinum
420218.6	with hemorrhage not confined to mediastinum (OIS Grade VI)
420499.3	**Brachiocephalic (innominate) artery** NFS (all OIS Grade III)
420402.3	intimal tear, no disruption
420404.3	laceration (perforation, puncture) NFS
420406.3	minor[i]
420408.4	major[j]
420699.3	**Branchiocephalic (innominate) vein,** NFS (all OIS Grade II)
420602.3	laceration (perforation, pucture) NFS
420604.3	minor[i]
420606.4	major[j]
420608.5	with air embolus right side
	Carotid artery (common, internal, external) see NECK
420800.5	**Coronary artery** laceration or thrombosis (left main, right main or left anterior descending artery; coronary sinus)
421099.3	**Pulmonary artery** NFS (all OIS Grades IV and V)
421002.3	intimal tear, no disruption
421004.3	laceration (perforation, puncture) NFS
421006.3	minor[i]
421008.4	major[j]
421299.3	**Pulmonary vein** NFS (all OIS Grades IV and V)
421202.3	laceration (perforation, puncture) NFS
421204.3	minor[i]
421206.4	major[j]
421499.3	**Subclavian artery** NFS (all OIS Grade III)
421402.3	intimal tear, no disruption
421404.3	laceration (perforation, puncture) NFS
421406.3	minor[i]
421408.4	major[j]

---

[i] superficial; incomplete transection; incomplete circumferential involvement; blood loss ≤20% by volume

[j] rupture; complete transection; segmental loss; complete circumferential involvement; blood loss >20% by volume

コード	損傷内容
420299.4	**胸部大動脈**　詳細不明
420202.4	内膜剥離（断裂なし）
420204.5	大動脈弁の損傷を伴う
420206.4	裂傷（穿孔，穿刺）　詳細不明
420208.4	小 [i]
420210.5	大 [j]
420212.5	大動脈基部または大動脈弁の損傷を伴う
420216.5	縦隔内に限局した出血を伴う
420218.6	縦隔外への出血を伴う（OIS Grade Ⅵ）
420499.3	**腕頭（無名）動脈**（すべて OIS Grade Ⅲ）詳細不明
420402.3	内膜剥離（断裂なし）
420404.3	裂傷（穿孔，穿刺）　詳細不明
420406.3	小 [i]
420408.4	大 [j]
420699.3	**腕頭（無名）静脈**（すべて OIS Grade Ⅱ）詳細不明
420602.3	裂傷（穿孔，穿刺）　詳細不明
420604.3	小 [i]
420606.4	大 [j]
420608.5	右心系の空気塞栓を伴う
	頸動脈（総頸，内頸，外頸）　頸部を参照
420800.5	**冠動脈**裂傷あるいは血栓症（左右冠動脈本幹あるいは前下行枝；冠静脈洞）
421099.3	**肺動脈**（すべて OIS Grade Ⅳ，Ⅴ）詳細不明
421002.3	内膜剥離（断裂なし）
421004.3	裂傷（穿孔，穿刺）　詳細不明
421006.3	小 [i]
421008.4	大 [j]
421299.3	**肺静脈**（すべて OIS Grade Ⅳ，Ⅴ）詳細不明
421202.3	裂傷（穿孔，穿刺）　詳細不明
421204.3	小 [i]
421206.4	大 [j]
421499.3	**鎖骨下動脈**（すべて OIS Grade Ⅲ）詳細不明
421402.3	内膜剥離（断裂なし）
421404.3	裂傷（穿孔，穿刺）　詳細不明
421406.3	小 [i]
421408.4	大 [j]

---

[i] 表在性；不完全断裂；非全周性；出血量が全血液量の20％以下。
[j] 破裂；完全断裂；部分欠損；全周性；出血量が全血液量の20％を超える。

THORAX

CODE	INJURY DESCRIPTION
421699.3	**Subclavian vein** NFS (all OIS Grade II)
421602.3	laceration (perforation, puncture) NFS
421604.3	minor[i]
421606.4	major[j]
421899.3	**Vena Cava, superior and thoracic portion of inferior,** NFS (OIS Grades IV and V)
421802.3	laceration (perforation, puncture) NFS
421804.3	minor with or without thrombosis[i]
421806.4	major[j]
421808.5	with air embolus right side
422099.2	**Other named arteries** NFS (e. g., bronchial, esophageal, intercostals, internal mammary) (all OIS Grade I)
422002.2	intimal tear, no disruption
422004.2	laceration (perforation, puncture) NFS
422006.2	minor[i]
422008.3	major[j]
422299.2	**Other named veins** NFS (e. g., azygos, bronchial, hemiazygus, intercostal, internal mammary, internal jugular) (all OIS Grade I except azygos, Grade II)
422202.2	laceration (perforation, puncture) NFS
422204.2	minor[i]
422206.3	major[j]

NERVES

Spinal cord see SPINE

Phrenic nerve see NECK

430499.1	**Vagus nerve** injury also see NECK and ABDOMEN

INTERNAL ORGANS

Bronchus, main stem see Trachea

440299.1	**Bronchus distal to main stem,** NFS
440202.1	contusion (hematoma)
440204.2	laceration (puncture) NFS
440206.2	no perforation; partial thickness
440208.3	perforation; full thickness but not complete transection
440210.4	complex; avulsion; rupture; transection
440212.3	fracture NFS
440214.3	simple
440216.4	major (with separation)

---

[i] superficial; incomplete transection; incomplete circumferential involvement; blood loss ≤20% by volume

[j] rupture; complete transection; segmental loss; complete circumferential involvement; blood loss >20% by volume

コード	損傷内容

421699.3　**鎖骨下静脈**（すべて OIS Grade Ⅱ）詳細不明
421602.3　　　　裂傷（穿孔，穿刺）詳細不明
421604.3　　　　　　小 ⁱ
421606.4　　　　　　大 ^j

421899.3　**上大静脈，胸腔内下大静脈**（OIS Grade Ⅳ，Ⅴ）詳細不明
421802.3　　　　裂傷（穿孔，穿刺）詳細不明
421804.3　　　　　　小 ⁱ　血栓の有無を問わない
421806.4　　　　　　大 ^j
421808.5　　　　　　　　　右心系の空気塞栓を伴う

422099.2　**その他の動脈**（例；気管支動脈，食道動脈，肋間動脈，内胸動脈）（すべて OIS Grade Ⅰ）詳細不明
422002.2　　　　内膜剥離（断裂なし）
422004.2　　　　裂傷（穿孔，穿刺）詳細不明
422006.2　　　　　　小 ⁱ
422008.3　　　　　　大 ^j

422299.2　**その他の静脈**（例；奇静脈，気管支静脈，半奇静脈，肋間静脈，内胸静脈，内頸静脈）（奇静脈はGrade Ⅱ，それ以外はすべて OIS Grade Ⅰ）詳細不明
422202.2　　　　裂傷（穿孔，穿刺）詳細不明
422204.2　　　　　　小 ⁱ
422206.3　　　　　　大 ^j

神経

　　　　脊髄　脊椎を参照
　　　　横隔神経　頸部を参照
430499.1　迷走神経損傷　頸部および腹部も参照

内臓

　　　　主気管支　気管の項を参照

440299.1　**主気管支より末梢の気管支**　詳細不明
440202.1　　　　挫傷（血腫）
440204.2　　　　裂傷・裂創（穿刺）詳細不明
440206.2　　　　　　穿孔なし；非全層性
440208.3　　　　　　穿孔あり；全層性であるが，完全断裂に至らない
440210.4　　　　　　複雑損傷；断裂；破裂；離断
440212.3　　　　軟骨骨折　詳細不明
440214.3　　　　　　単純
440216.4　　　　　　複雑（断裂を伴う）

ⁱ 表在性；不完全断裂；非全周性；出血量が全血液量の20％以下。
^j 破裂；完全断裂；部分欠損；全周性；出血量が全血液量の20％を超える。

THORAX

CODE	INJURY DESCRIPTION
440400.5	**Chordae tendinae** laceration (rupture)
440699.2	**Diaphragm** NFS
440602.2	contusion (OIS Grade I)
440604.3	laceration (OIS Grades II through IV)
440606.4	rupture with hernination
440899.2	**Esophagus** NFS
440802.2	contusion (hematoma)(Grade I)
440804.3	laceration NFS
440806.3	no perforation; partial thickness; ≤50% circumference (OIS Grades I and II)
440808.4	perforation; full thickness but not complete transection; >50% circumference (OIS Grade III)
440810.5	complex with tissue loss; avulsion; rupture; transection (OIS Grades IV, V)
441099.1	**Heart (Myocardium)** NFS
441002.1	contusion (hematoma) NFS
441004.1	minor — Patients presenting with dysrrthmia, wall motion abnormality, other ECG changes not related to CAD.
441006.4	major — This diagnosis must be substantiated e. g., by surgery, autopsy, EF <25% absent CAD.
441008.3	laceration NFS
441010.3	no perforation, no chamber involvement
441012.5	perforation (ventricular or atrial with or without tamponade)
441014.6	complex or ventricular rupture
441016.6	multiple lacerations; >50% tissue loss of a chamber
441018.6	avulsion
441200.5	**Intracardiac valve** laceration (rupture)
441300.5	**Interventricular** or **interatrial septum** laceration (rupture)
441499.3	**Lung** NFS
441402.3	contusion NFS
	This diagnosis should be coded only if there is history of chest trauma and a physician's diagnosis is documented by x-ray, CT, MRI, surgery or autopsy. Clinical pulmonary dysfunction is insufficient evidence of a codeable injury.
441406.3	unilateral — If associated with flail chest, see Flail Chest, page 25.
441410.4	bilateral

コード	損傷内容

440400.5　　腱索断裂（破裂）

440699.2　　横隔膜　詳細不明
440602.2　　　　　　挫傷（OIS Grade Ｉ）
440604.3　　　　　　裂傷・裂創（OIS Grade Ⅱ～Ⅳ）
440606.4　　　　　　ヘルニアを伴う破裂

440899.2　　食道　詳細不明
440802.2　　　　　挫傷（血腫）（OIS Grade Ｉ）
440804.3　　　　　裂傷・裂創　詳細不明
440806.3　　　　　　　　穿孔なし；非全層性，全周の50％以下の損傷（OIS Grade Ｉ，Ⅱ）
440808.4　　　　　　　　穿孔あり；全層性であるが，完全断裂に至らない；全周の50％を超える損傷
　　　　　　　　　　　　（OIS Grade Ⅲ）
440810.5　　　　　　　　組織欠損を伴う複雑損傷；断裂；破裂；離断（OIS Grade Ⅳ，Ⅴ）

441099.1　　心臓（心筋）　詳細不明
441002.1　　　　　挫傷（血腫）　詳細不明

441004.1　　　　　小　不整脈，壁運動異常および心電図変化（冠動脈疾患に関係しない）

441006.4　　　　　大　外科手術，剖検，EF25％以下（冠動脈疾患によらない）などが明らかな場合に限る。

441008.3　　　　　裂傷・裂創　詳細不明
441010.3　　　　　　　　穿孔なし，心房，心室損傷なし
441012.5　　　　　　　　穿孔あり（心室または心房の穿孔があるもので，タンポナーデの有無は問わない）
441014.6　　　　　　　　　　複雑損傷または心室の破裂
441016.6　　　　　　　　　　多発性裂傷；心房，心室の50％を超える組織欠損
441018.6　　　　　断裂

441200.5　　心臓弁裂傷・裂創（破裂）

441300.5　　心室または心房中隔の裂傷・裂創（破裂）

441499.3　　肺　詳細不明
441402.3　　　　　挫傷　詳細不明
　　　　　　　　　胸部外傷の病歴があり，かつⅩ線，CT，MRI，手術または剖検による医師の診断によって肺挫傷が認められた場合にのみこのコードを選択する。したがって，臨床的な肺機能障害だけでコードを選択することは不適当である。
441406.3　　　　　　　　片側　フレイルチェストに合併する場合は45ページ「フレイルチェスト」を参照
441410.4　　　　　　　　両側

THORAX

CODE	INJURY DESCRIPTION

Lung
    laceration

> If lung laceration coexists with rib fracture (s) and associated with hemo-/pneumothorax, code the hemo-/pneumothorax under the lung laceration only. Code the rib fracture (s) as if no hemo-/pneumothorax was present. Do not code the hemo-/pneumothorax separately.

Code	Description
441414.3	NFS with or without hemo-/pneumothorax unless described as follows:
441416.3	with pneumomediastinum
441418.4	with hemomediastinum
441420.4	with blood loss >20% by volume
441422.5	with tension pneumothorax
441424.5	with parenchymal laceration with massive air leak
441426.5	with systemic air embolus
441430.3	unilateral with or without hemo-/pneumothorax unless described as follows:
441432.3	with pneumomediastinum
441434.4	with hemomediastinum
441436.4	with blood loss >20% by volume
441438.5	with tension pneumothorax
441440.5	with parenchymal laceration with massive air leak
441442.5	with systemic air embolus
441450.4	bilateral with or without hemo-/pneumothorax unless described as follows:
441452.4	with pneumomediastinum
441454.4	with hemomediastinum
441456.5	with blood loss >20% by volume
441458.5	with tension pneumothorax
441460.5	with parenchymal laceration with massive air leak
441462.5	with systemic air embolus
441699.2	**Pericardium** NFS
441602.2	laceration (puncture)
441604.3	injury with tamponade without heart injury
441606.5	herniation of heart
441800.2	**Pleura** laceration
441802.3	with hemo-/pneumothorax

Pulmonary contusion   Code as Lung Contusion.

Code	Description
442999.9	**Thoracic cavity** injury NFS Use this section only when there is no information on specific anatomical lesion.
442202.3	with hemo-/pneumothorax
442204.3	with pneumomediastinum
442206.4	with hemomediastinum
442208.4	with blood loss >20% by volume
442210.5	with tension pneumothorax
442212.5	with systemic air embolism

コード	損傷内容

肺（続き）
　　裂傷

> 肺裂傷に肋骨骨折かつ血胸／気胸を合併している場合は，肺裂傷に血胸／気胸を加味してコードを選択する。そのさい肋骨骨折は血胸／気胸のないコードを選択する。血胸／気胸のコードを別に選択してはならない。

441414.3	詳細不明　血胸／気胸の有無は問わない（下記の場合を除く）
441416.3	縦隔気腫を伴う
441418.4	縦隔血腫を伴う
441420.4	出血量が全血液量の20％を超える
441422.5	緊張性気胸を伴う
441424.5	大量のエアリークと肺実質裂傷を伴う
441426.5	全身の空気塞栓を伴う
441430.3	片側性；血胸／気胸の有無は問わない（下記の場合を除く）
441432.3	縦隔気腫を伴う
441434.4	縦隔血腫を伴う
441436.4	出血量が全血液量の20％を超える
441438.5	緊張性気胸を伴う
441440.5	大量のエアリークと肺実質裂傷を伴う
441442.5	全身の空気塞栓を伴う
441450.4	両側性；血胸／気胸の有無は問わない（下記の場合を除く）
441452.4	縦隔気腫を伴う
441454.4	縦隔血腫を伴う
441456.5	出血量が全血液量の20％を超える
441458.5	緊張性気胸を伴う
441460.5	大量のエアリークと肺実質裂傷を伴う
441462.5	全身の空気塞栓を伴う

441699.2	**心膜（心嚢）**　詳細不明
441602.2	裂傷・裂創（穿刺）
441604.3	心損傷を伴わない心タンポナーデ
441606.5	心ヘルニア

| 441800.2 | **胸膜**裂傷・裂創 |
| 441802.3 | 　血胸／気胸を伴う |

| 442999.9 | **胸腔**損傷　詳細不明　　特定の解剖学的損傷の記載がない場合のみこのコードを選択する。 |

442202.3	血胸／気胸を伴う
442204.3	縦隔気腫を伴う
442206.4	縦隔血腫を伴う
442208.4	出血量が全血液量の20％を超える
442210.5	緊張性気胸を伴う
442212.5	全身の空気塞栓を伴う

THORAX

CODE	INJURY DESCRIPTION
442402.2	**Thoracic duct** laceration
442699.3	**Trachea and Main Stem Bronchus** NFS
442602.3	contusion (hematoma)
442604.3	laceration NFS
442606.3	no perforation; partial thickness
442608.4	perforation; full thickness but not complete transection
442610.5	complex, avulsion; rupture; transection
442612.4	fracture NFS
442614.4	simple
442616.5	major with laryngeal-tracheal separation

コード	損傷内容

442402.2　　**胸管**裂傷・裂創

442699.3　　**気管と主気管支**　詳細不明
442602.3　　　　　挫傷（血腫）
442604.3　　　　　裂傷　詳細不明
442606.3　　　　　　　穿孔なし；非全層性
442608.4　　　　　　　穿孔；全層性であるが，完全離断に至らない
442610.5　　　　　　　複雑損傷；断裂；破裂；離断
442612.4　　　　軟骨骨折　詳細不明
442614.4　　　　　　　単純
442616.5　　　　　　　複雑（喉頭と気管の分離を伴う）

THORAX

CODE	INJURY DESCRIPTION

SKELETAL

450299.1	**Rib cage** NFS
450202.1	contusion
450210.2	multiple rib fractures NFS Use this code if no other information available.

> If rib fracture (s) coexist with lung laceration (s) <u>and</u> are associated with hemo-/pneumothorax, code the hemo-/pneumothorax under the lung injury only. Code the rib fracture (s) as if no hemo-/pneumothorax were present. Do not code the hemo-/pneumothorax separately.

450211.3	with hemo-/pneumothorax
450212.1	1 rib
450214.3	with hemo-/pneumothorax (OIS Grade I)
450220.2	2-3 ribs any location or multiple fractures of single rib, with stable chest or NFS (OIS Grade I, II, III)
450222.3	with hemo-/pneumothorax
450230.3	>3 ribs on one side and no more than 3 ribs on other side, stable chest or NFS
450232.4	with hemo-/pneumothorax
450240.4	>3 ribs on each of two sides, with stable chest or NFS
450242.5	with hemo-/pneumothorax
450250.3	open/displaced/comminuted any or combination (≥1 rib)
450252.4	with hemo-/pneumothorax
450260.3	flail chest, (unstable chest wall, paradoxical chest movement) unilateral or NFS (OIS Grade III or IV)
450262.3	without lung contusion (OIS Grade III or IV)
450264.4	with lung contusion (OIS Grade III or IV)
450266.5	bilateral (OIS Grade V)

> If tension pneumothorax occurs with rib fractures but no documented lung injury, tension PTX should be coded separately under "Thoracic cavity injury with tension PTX" 442210.5 and the rib fractures should be coded with no PTX.

450899.1	**Sternum** NFS
450802.1	contusion
450804.2	fracture (OIS Grade II or III)

コード	損傷内容

骨　格

450299.1	**肋骨**	詳細不明
450202.1		挫傷

450210.2　　　　　多発肋骨骨折　詳細不明　これ以上の情報が得られなければこのコードを選択する。

> 肋骨骨折に肺裂傷かつ血胸／気胸を合併している場合は，肺裂傷に血胸／気胸を加味してコードを選択する。そのさい肋骨骨折は血胸／気胸のないコードを選択する。血胸／気胸のコードを別に選択してはならない。

450211.3	血胸／気胸を伴う
450212.1	1本の肋骨骨折
450214.3	血胸，気胸を伴う（OIS Grade Ⅰ）
450220.2	2～3本の肋骨骨折，または1本の肋骨骨折（複数部位），ただし胸郭動揺はないか不明（OIS Grade Ⅰ，Ⅱ，Ⅲ）
450222.3	血胸／気胸を伴う
450230.3	一側が4本以上の肋骨骨折，反対側は3本以下，ただし胸郭動揺はないか不明
450232.4	血胸／気胸を伴う
450240.4	両側が4本以上の肋骨骨折，胸壁動揺がないか不明
450242.5	血胸／気胸を伴う
450250.3	開放／転位／粉砕　いずれか1つ以上　（本数は問わず）
450252.4	血胸／気胸を伴う
450260.3	フレイルチェスト（不安定胸郭，奇異性胸郭運動），片側性または詳細不明（OIS Grade ⅢあるいはⅣ）
450262.3	肺挫傷を伴わない（OIS Grade ⅢあるいはⅣ）
450264.4	肺挫傷を伴う（OIS Grade ⅢあるいはⅣ）
450266.5	両側（OIS Grade Ⅴ）

> 肋骨骨折に伴う緊張性気胸で，肺損傷が記載されていない場合，緊張性気胸は「胸腔損傷の緊張性気胸」442210.5のコードを選択し，肋骨骨折は気胸のないコードを選択する。

450899.1	**胸骨**	詳細不明
450802.1		挫傷
450804.2		骨折（OIS GradeⅡあるいはⅢ）

腹部および骨盤内臓器

ABDOMEN AND PELVIC CONTENTS

CODE	INJURY DESCRIPTION

WHOLE AREA

516000.1	**Penetrating injury** NFS
516002.1	superficial; minor; into peritoneum but not involving deeper structures
516004.2	with tissue loss $>100cm^2$ but blood loss $<20\%$ by volume
516006.3	with blood loss $>20\%$ by volume

> If deeper structures are involved, code under Vessels or Organs.

> Assign one of the following codes, as appropriate, to soft tissue injuries to the abdomen. To calculate an ISS, however, assign injuries in this category to the External body region and follow rules for ISS calculation on pages xviii and xix.

510099.1	**Skin/Subcutaneous/muscle** NFS
510202.1	abrasion
510402.1	contusion (hematoma)
510600.1	laceration
510602.1	minor; superficial
510604.2	major ($>20cm$ long and into subcutaneous tissue)
510606.3	blood loss $>20\%$ by volume
510800.1	avulsion NFS
510802.1	minor; superficial; ($<100cm^2$)
510804.2	major ($>100cm^2$ but blood loss $<20\%$ by volume)
510806.3	blood loss $>20\%$ by volume

> Use one of the following two descriptors when such vague information is the only description available. These descriptors allow a means for identifying the occurrence of abdominal injury, but they do not allow the calculation of an accurate ISS in these patients.

515099.9	**Blunt/traumatic abdominal injury** NFS
515999.9	Died without further evaluation; no autopsy

VESSELS

> Vessel injuries are coded as separate injuries if: (1) they are isolated injuries (i. e., no accompanying documented organ injury) or (2) accompanying organ injury does not include any vessel injury description or (3) named vessel injury occurs with organ injury and is higher in severity than descriptor for organ injury.
> The terms "laceration", "puncture" and "perforation" are oftentimes used interchangeably to describe vessel injuries. When "perforation" or "puncture" is used, code as laceration. Descriptions for vessel lacerations distinguish between complete and incomplete transection. See footnotes "i" and "j".

腹部および骨盤内臓器

コード	損傷内容

全 域

516000.1	**穿通性損傷**　詳細不明
516002.1	表在性；小；腹膜に達するが，深部組織の損傷は伴わない
516004.2	組織欠損が100cm^{2}を超えるが，出血量が全血液量の20％以下
516006.3	出血量が全血液量の20％を超える

> 深部組織の損傷を伴う場合は，「血管」または「内臓」のコードを選択する。

> 腹部への軟部組織損傷には，以下のコードの中の適切なものを選択する。ただし ISS を算出する場合には，「腹部」ではなく「体表」の区分として取り扱い，21，22ページの ISS 計算ルールに従う。

510099.1	**皮膚／皮下組織／筋肉**　詳細不明
510202.1	擦過傷
510402.1	挫傷（血腫）
510600.1	裂創
510602.1	小；表在性
510604.2	大（長さが20cm を超え，かつ皮下組織に達する）
510606.3	出血量が全血液量の20％を超える
510800.1	剥離　詳細不明
510802.1	小；表在性；（100cm^{2}以下）
510804.2	大（100cm^{2}を超えるが，出血量は全血液量の20％以下）
510806.3	出血量が全血液量の20％を超える

> 不確定な情報しか得られない場合には，以下の2つのコードのうちいずれかを選択する。ただしこれらのコードを選択した場合には ISS は計算してはならない。

515099.9	**鈍的腹部損傷**　詳細不明
515999.9	死亡（詳細な評価なし）；剖検なし

血 管

> 血管損傷は，以下の場合には独立した傷害としてコードを選択する。
> (1)単独血管損傷（臓器損傷がない血管損傷）
> (2)臓器損傷に血管損傷に関する記載がないとき
> (3)血管損傷と臓器損傷が合併していて，血管損傷の重症度が臓器損傷の重症度より高いとき
> 血管損傷を表わす場合，"裂傷""穿刺""穿孔"などの用語はしばしば同じような意味で用いられる。血管の"穿孔"や"穿刺"と記載されている場合は"裂傷"としてコード選択する。血管の裂傷については，完全断裂と不全断裂に区分する。脚注 i, j を参照。

ABDOMEN AND PELVIC CONTENTS

CODE	INJURY DESCRIPTION
520299.4	**Aorta, Abdominal** NFS
520202.4	intimal tear, no disruption
520204.4	laceration (perforation, puncture) NFS
520206.4	minor[i]
520208.5	major[j]
520499.3	**Celiac Artery** NFS
520402.3	intimal tear, no disruption
520404.3	laceration (perforation, puncture) NFS
520406.4	minor[i]
520408.5	major[j]
520699.3	**Iliac artery (common, internal, external)** NFS
520602.3	intimal tear, no disruption
520604.3	laceration (perforation, puncture) NFS
520606.3	minor[i]
520608.4	major[j]
520899.3	**Iliac vein (common)** NFS
520802.3	laceration (perforation, puncture) NFS
520804.3	minor[i]
520806.4	major[j]
521099.2	**Iliac vein (internal, external)** NFS
521002.2	laceration (perforation, puncture) NFS
521004.2	minor[i] with or without thrombosis
521006.3	major[j]
521299.3	Vena cava, inferior, NFS
521202.3	laceration (perforation, puncture) NFS
521204.3	minor[i] with or without thrombosis
521206.4	major[j]
	Vena cava, retrohepatic see Liver
521499.3	**Other named arteries** NFS (e. g., hepatic, renal, splenic, superior mesenteric)
521402.3	intimal tear, no disruption
521404.3	laceration (perforation, puncture) NFS
521406.3	minor[i]
521408.4	major[j]
521699.3	**Other named veins** NFS (e. g., portal, renal, splenic, superior mesenteric)
521602.3	laceration (perforation, puncture) NFS
521604.3	minor[i] with or without thrombosis
521606.4	major[j]

[i] superficial; incomplete transection; incomplete circumferential involvement; blood loss ≤20% by volume
[j] rupture; complete transection; segmental loss; complete circumferential involvement; blood loss >20% by volume

腹部および骨盤内臓器

コード	損傷内容
520299.4	**腹部大動脈**　詳細不明
520202.4	内膜剥離（断裂なし）
520204.4	裂傷（穿孔，穿刺）　詳細不明
520206.4	小 [i]
520208.5	大 [j]
520499.3	**腹腔動脈**　詳細不明
520402.3	内膜剥離（断裂なし）
520404.3	裂傷（穿孔，穿刺）　詳細不明
520406.4	小 [i]
520408.5	大 [j]
520699.3	**腸骨動脈（総，内，外）**　詳細不明
520602.3	内膜剥離（断裂なし）
520604.3	裂傷（穿孔，穿刺）　詳細不明
520606.3	小 [i]
520608.4	大 [j]
520899.3	**総腸骨静脈**　詳細不明
520802.3	裂傷（穿孔，穿刺）　詳細不明
520804.3	小 [i]
520806.4	大 [j]
521099.2	**腸骨静脈（内，外）**　詳細不明
521002.2	裂傷（穿孔，穿刺）　詳細不明
521004.2	小 [i]　血栓の有無を問わない
521006.3	大 [j]
521299.3	**下大静脈**　詳細不明
521202.3	裂傷（穿孔，穿刺）　詳細不明
521204.3	小 [i]　血栓の有無を問わない
521206.4	大 [j]
	下大静脈（肝後面） 　肝臓の項を参照
521499.3	**その他の動脈**（例；肝動脈，腎動脈，脾動脈，上腸間膜動脈）詳細不明
521402.3	内膜剥離（断裂なし）
521404.3	裂傷（穿孔，穿刺）　詳細不明
521406.3	小 [i]
521408.4	大 [j]
521699.3	**その他の静脈**（例；門脈，腎静脈，脾静脈，上腸間膜静脈）詳細不明
521602.3	裂傷（穿孔，穿刺）　詳細不明
521604.3	小 [i]　血栓の有無を問わない
521606.4	大 [j]

---

[i] 表在性；不完全断裂；非全周性；出血量が全血液量の20％以下。
[j] 破裂；完全断裂；部分欠損；全周性；出血量が全血液量の20％を超える。

ABDOMEN AND PELVIC CONTENTS

CODE	INJURY DESCRIPTION

NERVES

       Lumbar spinal cord see SPINE

       Cauda equina see SPINE

530499.1   **Vagus nerve** injury also see NECK & THORAX

INTERNAL ORGANS

Code	Description
540299.1	**Adrenal gland** NFS
540210.1	contusion (hematoma) NFS
540212.1	minor; superficial
540214.2	major; large; deep
540220.1	laceration NFS
540222.1	minor; superficial
540224.2	major; multiple lacerations
540226.3	massive; avulsion; complex; rupture; stellate; tissue loss; blood loss >20% by volume
540499.1	**Anus** NFS
540410.1	contusion (hematoma)
540420.2	laceration NFS
540422.2	no perforation; partial thickness
540424.3	perforation; full thickness but not complete transection
540426.4	massive; avulsion; complex; rupture; tissue loss
540699.2	**Bladder** (urinary) NFS
540610.2	contusion (hematoma) (OIS Grade I)
540620.2	laceration NFS
540622.3	no perforation; partial thickness (OIS Grade I)
540624.4	perforation; full thickness but not complete transection (OIS Grades II, III, IV)
540626.4	massive; avulsion; complex; tissue loss (OIS Grades II, III, IV)
540640.3	rupture NFS Use this code only when a more detailed description is not available.
540899.2	**Colon** (large bowel) NFS
540810.2	contusion (hematoma) (OIS Grade I)
540820.2	laceration NFS
540822.2	no perforation; partial thickness; <50% of circumference (OIS Grades I and II)
540824.3	perforation; full thickness; ≥50% of circumference without transection (OIS Grade III)
540826.4	massive; avulsion; complex; rupture; tissue loss; gross fecal contamination; transection; devascularization (OIS Grades IV and V)

コード	損傷内容

神 経

    腰髄　脊椎を参照

    馬尾　脊椎を参照

530499.1 迷走神経損傷　頸部および胸部も参照

内 臓

540299.1 副腎　詳細不明
540210.1   挫傷（血腫）　詳細不明
540212.1   小；表在性
540214.2   大；大きい；深い
540220.1   裂傷・裂創　詳細不明
540222.1   小；表在性
540224.2   大；多発性裂傷・裂創
540226.3   広範囲；断裂；複雑；破裂；粉砕；組織欠損；出血量が全血液量の20％を超える

540499.1 肛門　詳細不明
540410.1   挫傷（血腫）
540420.2   裂傷・裂創　詳細不明
540422.2   穿孔なし；非全層性
540424.3   穿孔あり；全層性であるが，完全断裂には至らない
540426.4   広範囲；断裂；複雑；破裂；組織欠損

540699.2 膀胱　詳細不明
540610.2   挫傷（血腫）（OIS Grade Ⅰ）
540620.2   裂傷・裂創　詳細不明
540622.3   穿孔なし；非全層性（OIS Grade Ⅰ）
540624.4   穿孔あり；全層性であるが，完全断裂には至らない（OIS Grade Ⅱ，Ⅲ，Ⅳ）
540626.4   広範囲；断裂；複雑；組織欠損（OIS Grade Ⅱ，Ⅲ，Ⅳ）
540640.3   破裂　詳細不明　より詳細な情報のない場合にのみこのコードを選択する。

540899.2 結腸（大腸）　詳細不明
540810.2   挫傷（血腫）（OIS Grade Ⅰ）
540820.2   裂傷・裂創　詳細不明
540822.2   穿孔なし；非全層性；周径の50％未満の裂傷（OIS Grade ⅠおよびⅡ）
540824.3   穿孔あり；全層性；周径の50％以上であるが完全断裂には至らない（OIS Grade Ⅲ）
540826.4   広範囲；断裂；複雑；破裂；組織欠損；糞便による汚染；離断；血行遮断
        （OIS Grade ⅣおよびⅤ）

ABDOMEN AND PELVIC CONTENTS

CODE	INJURY DESCRIPTION

541099.2　**Duodenum** NFS
541010.2　　　contusion (hematoma) (OIS Grades I or II)
541020.2　　　laceration NFS
541022.2　　　　　disruption <50% of circumference; no perforation; partial thickness; serosal tear (OIS Grades I or II)

541023.3　　　　　disruption 50-75% circumference of D2^L; disruption 50-100% circumference of D1, D3, D4^L (OIS Grade III)

541024.4　　　　　disruption >75% circumference of D2^L; involving ampulla or destal common bile duct (OIS Grade IV)

541028.5　　　　　massive; avulsion; complex; rupture; tissue loss; gross enteric contamination; devascularization; massive disruption of duodenopancreatic complex (OIS Grade V)

　　　　Esophagus see THORAX

　　　　Cystic duct injury see Gallbladder

541299.2　**Gallbladder** NFS
541210.2　　　contusion (hematoma) (OIS Grade I)
541220.2　　　laceration, (perforation) NFS (OIS Grade II)
541222.2　　　　　minor; superficial; no cystic duct involvement

541224.3　　　　　massive; avulsion; complex; rupture; tissue loss; cystic duct laceration or transection^m (OIS Grade III)
541226.4　　　　　　　with common bile or hepatic duct laceration or transection^m (OIS Grades IV and V)

541499.2　**Jejunum-ileum** (small bowel) NFS
541410.2　　　contusion (hematoma) (OIS Grade I)
541420.2　　　laceration NFS
541422.2　　　　　no perforation; partial thickness; <50% of circumference (OIS Grade I or II)

541424.3　　　　　perforation; full thickness; ≥50% of circumference without transection (OIS Grade III)

541426.4　　　　　massive; avulsion; complex; rupture; tissue loss; transection; devascularization (OIS Grade IV or V)

541699.2　**Kidney** NFS
541610.2　　　contusion (hematoma) NFS
541612.2　　　　　subcapsular, nonexpanding confined to renal retroperitoneum or without parenchymal laceration; minor; superficial; (OIS Grade I or II)

541614.3　　　　　subcapsular; >50% surface area or expanding; major; large

---

^{L} D1= superior or first part; D2= descending or second part; D3 = horizontal or third part; D4 = ascending or fourth part
^{m} "Duct involvement" applies only to gallbladder, liver and pancreas. Injuries to these organs, which really share the same duct system, not infrequently involve injuries to the duct systems of each organ. When there is one ductal injury, it should be assigned to either (not both) of the two involved organs. On the other hand, when separate ductal injuries (e. g., to the right hepatic duct and the pancreatic duct) occur, they should be assigned to both organs.

腹部および骨盤内臓器

コード	損傷内容

541099.2　十二指腸　詳細不明
541010.2　　　　挫傷（血腫）（OIS Grade ⅠまたはⅡ）
541020.2　　　　裂傷・裂創　詳細不明
541022.2　　　　　　周径の50％未満；穿孔なし；非全層性；漿膜裂傷（OIS GradeⅠまたはⅡ）

541023.3　　　　　　D2^{L}の周径の50〜75％；D1，D3，D4^{L}の周径の50〜100％（OIS Grade Ⅲ）

541024.4　　　　　　D2^{L}の周径の75％を超える；膨大部または遠位総胆管の損傷を合併する
　　　　　　　　　　（OIS Grade Ⅳ）

541028.5　　　　　　広範囲；断裂；複雑；破裂；組織欠損；腸内容による高度の汚染；血行遮断；十二指腸・膵臓結合部の高度の損傷（OIS Grade Ⅴ）

　　　　食道　胸部を参照
　　　　胆嚢管損傷　胆嚢の項を参照

541299.2　胆嚢　詳細不明
541210.2　　　挫傷（血腫）（OIS Grade Ⅰ）
541220.2　　　裂傷・裂創，（穿孔）（OIS Grade Ⅱ）詳細不明
541222.2　　　　　小；表在性；胆嚢管の損傷なし

541224.3　　　　　広範囲；断裂；複雑；破裂；組織欠損；胆嚢管の裂傷・裂創または離断^m（OIS Grade Ⅲ）

541226.4　　　　　　総胆管または肝管の裂傷・裂創または離断を伴う^m（OIS Grade Ⅳおよび Ⅴ）

541499.2　空腸—回腸（小腸）　詳細不明
541410.2　　　挫傷（血腫）（OIS Grade Ⅰ）
541420.2　　　裂傷・裂創　詳細不明
541422.2　　　　穿孔なし；非全層性；周径の50％未満の裂傷（OIS GradeⅠまたはⅡ）

541424.3　　　　穿孔あり；全層性；周径の50％以上であるが完全断裂には至らない
　　　　　　　　（OIS Grade Ⅲ）

541426.4　　　　広範囲；断裂；複雑；破裂；組織欠損；離断；血行遮断
　　　　　　　　（OIS Grade ⅣまたはⅤ）

541699.2　腎臓　詳細不明
541610.2　　　挫傷（血腫）　詳細不明
541612.2　　　　被膜下；腎周囲に限局；実質の裂傷なし；小；表在性；（OIS GradeⅠまたはⅡ）

541614.3　　　　被膜下；表面積の50％を超える；腎周囲を越える；大；広範囲

---

^{L} D1は上部または第1部；D2は下行部または第2部；D3は水平部または第3部；D4は上行部または第4部。
^{m}「管路の損傷の合併」は胆嚢，肝臓，膵臓にのみ適用される。これらの臓器は，実際は同じ導管系を共有しているので，各臓器にまたがる導管系の傷害となることが少なくない。1つの管路の損傷の場合，その管路系に関係する2つの臓器のいずれか一方にコードを記入する。これに対し，別の2つの管路に損傷が発生した場合（例えば，右肝管と膵管の損傷），両方の臓器のコードを選択する。

ABDOMEN AND PELVIC CONTENTS

CODE	INJURY DESCRIPTION
	Kidney (continued)
541620.2	laceration NFS
541622.2	<1cm parenchymal depth of renal cortex without urinary extravasation; minor; superficial; (OIS Grade II)
541624.3	>1cm parenchymal depth of renal cortex without collecting system rupture or urinary extravasation; moderate; (OIS Grade III)
541626.4	extending through renal cortex, medulla and collecting system; main renal vessel injury with contained hemorrhage; major; (OIS Grade IV)
541628.5	hilum avulsion; total destruction of organ and its vascular system (OIS Grade V)
541640.4	rupture Use this code only when a more detailed description is not available.
541899.2	**Liver** NFS
541810.2	contusion (hematoma) NFS
541812.2	subcapsular, ≤50% surface area, nonexpanding or intraparenchymal ≤10cm in diameter; minor; superficial; (OIS Grade I or II)
541814.3	>50% surface area or expanding; ruptured subcapsular or parenchymal; intraparenchymal >10cm or expanding; blood loss >20% by volume; major; subcapsular; (OIS Grade III)
541820.2	laceration NFS
541822.2	simple capsular tears, ≤3cm parenchymal depth, ≤10cm in length; blood loss ≤20% by volume; minor; superficial (OIS Grade I or II)
541824.3	>3cm parenchymal depth; major duct involvement[m]; blood loss >20% by volume; moderate (OIS Grade III)
541826.4	parenchymal disruption of ≤75% of hepatic lobe or 1-3 Couinaud's segments within a single lobe; multiple lacerations >3cm deep; "burst" injury; major (OIS Grade IV)
541828.5	parenchymal disruption of >75% of hepatic lobe or involving >3 Couinard's segments within a single lobe or involving retrohepatic vena cava/central hepatic veins; massive; complex; (OIS Grade V)
541830.6	hepatic avulsion (total separation of all vascular attachments) (OIS Grade VI)
541840.4	rupture ("fracture") NFS Use this code only when a more detailed description is not available.

[m] "Duct involvement" applies only to gallbladder, liver and pancreas. Injuries to these organs, which really share the same duct system, not infrequently involve injuries to the duct systems of each organ. When there is one ductal injury, it should be assigned to either (not both) of the two involved organs. On the other hand, when separate ductal injuries (e.g., to the right hepatic duct and the pancreatic duct) occur, they should be assigned to both organs.

コード	損傷内容
	腎臓（続き）
541620.2	裂傷・裂創　詳細不明
541622.2	深さ1cm以下の腎皮質実質の損傷，溢尿なし；小；表在性；（OIS Grade Ⅱ）
541624.3	深さ1cmを超える腎皮質実質の損傷，腎盂腎杯の破裂，溢尿なし；中；（OIS Grade Ⅲ）
541626.4	腎皮質を貫通し，髄質，腎盂腎杯に達する損傷；腎茎部の血管損傷で出血を伴う；大；（OIS Grade Ⅳ）
541628.5	腎門部の断裂；腎組織および血管系の高度の損傷（OIS Grade Ⅴ）
541640.4	破裂　より詳細な情報のない場合にのみこのコードを選択する。
541899.2	**肝臓**　詳細不明
541810.2	挫傷（血腫）　詳細不明
541812.2	被膜下；表面積の50％以下；限局性；直径10cm以内；小；表在性；（OIS Grade ⅠまたはⅡ）
541814.3	表面積の50％を超える；非限局性；被膜下または実質の破裂；直径10cmを超える；出血量が全血液量の20％を超える；大；被膜下；（OIS Grade Ⅲ）
541820.2	裂傷・裂創　詳細不明
541822.2	単純な被膜裂傷・裂創，実質の深さ3cm以下，長さ10cm以下；出血量が全血液量の20％以下；小；表在性（OIS Grade ⅠまたはⅡ）
541824.3	実質の深さ3cmを超える；胆道損傷を合併[m]；出血量が全血液量の20％を超える；中等度（OIS Grade Ⅲ）
541826.4	一葉の1～3クイノー肝区域または75％以下の実質の損傷；深さ3cm以上の多発性裂傷；"破裂"；大（OIS Grade Ⅳ）
541828.5	一葉の4以上のクイノー肝区域または75％を超える実質の損傷，肝後面下大静脈もしくは肝静脈の損傷を伴う実質の損傷；広範囲；複雑；（OIS Grade Ⅴ）
541830.6	肝断裂（肝血管系の完全分離）（OIS Grade Ⅵ）
541840.4	破裂（"fracture"）　詳細不明　より詳細な情報のない場合にのみこのコードを選択する。

---

[m]「管路の損傷の合併」は胆嚢，肝臓，膵臓にのみ適用される。これらの臓器は，実際は同じ導管系を共有しているので，各臓器にまたがる導管系の傷害となることが少なくない。1つの管路の損傷の場合，その管系に関係する2つの臓器のいずれか一方にコードを記入する。これに対し，別の2つの管路に損傷が発生した場合（例えば，右肝管と膵管の損傷），両方の臓器のコードを選択する。

ABDOMEN AND PELVIC CONTENTS

CODE	INJURY DESCRIPTION

542099.2 **Mesentery** NFS
542010.2   contusion (hematoma)
542020.2   laceration NFS
542022.2   minor; superficial
542024.3   major; blood loss >20% by volume
542026.4   massive; avulsion; complex; rupture; stellate; tissue loss

542299.2 **Omentum** NFS
542210.2   contusion (hematoma)
542220.2   laceration NFS
542222.2   minor; superficial
542224.3   major; blood loss >20% by volume

542400.2 **Ovarian (Fallopian) tube** laceration

542699.1 **Ovary** NFS
542610.1   contusion (hematoma) (OIS Grade I)
542620.2   laceration (perforation) NFS
542622.2   ≤ .5cm; minor; superficial (OIS Grade II)
542624.3   deep; > .5cm; complete parenchymal destruction; partial disruption of blood supply; massive; avulsion; complex; rupture (OIS Grades III, IV, V)

542899.2 **Pancreas** NFS
542810.2   contusion (hematoma)
542812.2   minor; superficial; no duct involvement (OIS Grade I)
542814.3   major; large; extensive; duct involvement (OIS Grade I or II)
542820.2   laceration NFS
542822.2   minor; superficial; no duct involvement (OIS Grade I)
542824.3   moderate; with major vessel or major duct involvement[m] (OIS Grade III)
542826.4   if involving ampulla (OIS Grade IV)
542828.4   major; multiple lacerations
542830.4   if involving ampulla (OIS Grade IV)
542832.5   massive; avulsion; complex; rupture; stellate; tissue loss; massive disruption of pancreatic head (OIS Grade V)

543099.1 **Penis** NFS
543010.1   contusion (hematoma)
543020.1   laceration (perforation) NFS
543022.1   minior; superficial
543024.2   major
543026.3   massive; amputation; avulsion; complex; rupture

543299.1 **Perineum** NFS
543210.1   contusion (hematoma)
543220.1   laceration (perforation) NFS
543222.1   minor; superficial
543224.2   major
543226.3   massive; avulsion; complex; rupture

---

[m] "Duct involvement" applies only to gallbladder, liver and pancreas. Injuries to these organs, which really share the same duct system, not infrequently involve injuries to the duct systems of each organ. When there is one ductal injury, it should be assigned to either (not both) of the two involved organs. On the other hand, when separate ductal injuries (e. g., to the right hepatic duct and the pancreatic duct) occur, they should be assigned to both organs.

コード	損傷内容
542099.2	**腸間膜** 詳細不明
542010.2	挫傷（血腫）
542020.2	裂傷・裂創　詳細不明
542022.2	小；表在性
542024.3	大；出血量が全血液量の20％を超える
542026.4	広範囲；断裂；複雑；破裂；粉砕；組織欠損
542299.2	**大網** 詳細不明
542210.2	挫傷（血腫）
542220.2	裂傷・裂創　詳細不明
542222.2	小；表在性
542224.3	大；出血量が全血液量の20％を超える
542400.2	**卵管（ファロピアン管）** 裂傷・裂創
542699.1	**卵巣** 詳細不明
542610.1	挫傷（血腫）（OIS Grade Ⅰ）
542620.2	裂傷・裂創（穿孔）　詳細不明
542622.2	0.5cm 以下；小；表在性（OIS Grade Ⅱ）
542624.3	深在性；0.5cmを超える；実質の完全破壊；部分的な血行遮断；広範囲；断裂；複雑；破裂（OIS Grade Ⅲ，Ⅳ，Ⅴ）
542899.2	**膵臓** 詳細不明
542810.2	挫傷（血腫）
542812.2	小；表在性；膵管の損傷なし（OIS Grade Ⅰ）
542814.3	大；大きい；広範囲；膵管の損傷を伴う（OIS Grade Ⅰ またはⅡ）
542820.2	裂傷・裂創　詳細不明
542822.2	小；表在性；膵管の損傷なし（OIS Grade Ⅰ）
542824.3	中；大血管または主膵管の損傷を伴う[m]（OIS Grade Ⅲ）
542826.4	膨大部の損傷を伴う（OIS Grade Ⅳ）
542828.4	大；多発性裂傷
542830.4	膨大部の損傷を伴う（OIS Grade Ⅳ）
542832.5	広範囲；断裂；複雑；破裂；粉砕；組織欠損；膵頭部の高度の損傷（OIS Grade Ⅴ）
543099.1	**陰茎** 詳細不明
543010.1	挫傷（血腫）
543020.1	裂傷・裂創（穿孔）　詳細不明
543022.1	小；表在性
543024.2	大
543026.3	広範囲；切断；断裂；複雑；破裂
543299.1	**会陰部** 詳細不明
543210.1	挫傷（血腫）
543220.1	裂傷・裂創（穿孔）　詳細不明
543222.1	小；表在性
543224.2	大
543226.3	広範囲；断裂；複雑；破裂

---

[m]「管路の損傷の合併」は胆嚢，肝臓，膵臓にのみ適用される。これらの臓器は，実際は同じ導管系を共有しているので，各臓器にまたがる導管系の傷害となることが少なくない。1つの管路の損傷の場合，その管路系に関係する2つの臓器のいずれか一方にコードを記入する。これに対し，別の2つの管路に損傷が発生した場合（例えば，右肝管と膵管の損傷），両方の臓器のコードを選択する。

ABDOMEN AND PELVIC CONTENTS

CODE	INJURY DESCRIPTION
543400.3	**Placenta** abruption NFS
543402.4	blood loss >20% by volume
543699.2	**Rectum** NFS
543610.2	contusion (hematoma) (OIS Grade I)
543620.2	laceration NFS
543622.2	no perforation; partial thickness; <50% of circumference (OIS Grades I and II)
543624.3	full thickness; ≥50% of circumference (OIS Grade III)
543625.4	full thickness extending into perineum (OIS Grade IV)
543626.5	massive; avulsion; complex; rupture; tissue loss; devascularization; gross fecal contamination of pelvic space (OIS Grade V)
543800.3	**Retroperitoneum** hemorrhage or hematoma

> If this injury occurs in combination with other thoracic or abdominal injury, code it separately using this description <u>only</u> if it can be determined that it is unrelated to the other injury. This description may also be used when no anatomical injury has been documented.
>
> The following organs or structures, when injured, may cause retroperitoneal hemorrhage: pancreas, duodenum, kidney, aorta, vena cava, mesenteric vessel; also pelvic or vertebral fractures.

544099.1	**Scrotum** NFS
544010.1	contusion (hematoma)
544020.1	laceration (perforation) NFS
544022.1	minor; superficial
544024.2	major; amputation; avulsion; complex
544299.2	**Spleen** NFS
544210.2	contusion (hematoma) NFS
544212.2	subcapsular, ≤50% surface area; intraparenchymal, nonexpanding, <5cm in diameter; minor; superficial; (OIS Grade I or II)
544214.3	subcapsular, >50% surface area or expanding; ruptured subcapsular or parenchymal; intraparenchymal >5cm in diameter or expanding; major; (OIS Grade III)
544220.2	laceration NFS
544222.2	simple capsular tear ≤3cm parenchymal depth; no major (i. e., trabecular) vessel involvement; minor; superficial; (OIS Grade I or II)
544224.3	no hilar or segmental parenchymal disruption or destruction; >3cm parenchymal depth or involving major (i. e., trabecular) vessels; moderate (OIS Grade III)
544226.4	involving segmental or hilar vessels producing major devascularization of >25% of spleen but no hilar injury; major (OIS Grade IV)
544228.5	hilar disruption producing total devascularization: tissue loss; avulsion; stellate; massive; (OIS Grade V)

コード	損傷内容

543400.3　**胎盤**剝離　詳細不明
543402.4　　　　　出血量が全血液量の20％を超える

543699.2　**直腸**　詳細不明
543610.2　　　　　挫傷（血腫）（OIS Grade Ⅰ）
543620.2　　　　　裂傷・裂創　詳細不明
543622.2　　　　　　　穿孔なし；非全層性；周径の50％未満（OIS Grade Ⅰ および Ⅱ）

543624.3　　　　　　　全層性；周径の50％以上（OIS Grade Ⅲ）
543625.4　　　　　　　全層性，会陰部に達する（OIS Grade Ⅳ）

543626.5　　　　　　　広範囲；断裂；複雑；破裂；組織欠損；血行遮断；
　　　　　　　　　　　骨盤腔の糞便による高度汚染（OIS Grade Ⅴ）

543800.3　**後腹膜**出血または血腫

> 後腹膜出血が胸部または腹部損傷と同時に存在している場合は，これらの損傷と無関係のときにのみ独立してコードを選択する。このコードは，損傷部位の解剖学的記載がない場合でも使用できる。
>
> 次の損傷は，後腹膜出血の原因となる：膵臓，十二指腸，腎臓，大動脈，大静脈，腸間膜血管；または骨盤，脊椎の骨折

544099.1　**陰嚢**　詳細不明
544010.1　　　　　挫傷（血腫）
544020.1　　　　　裂傷・裂創（穿孔）　詳細不明
544022.1　　　　　　　小；表在性
544024.2　　　　　　　大；切断；断裂；複雑

544299.2　**脾臓**　詳細不明
544210.2　　　　　挫傷（血腫）　詳細不明
544212.2　　　　　　　被膜下，表面積の50％以下；実質内，限局性，直径5 cm以下；小；
　　　　　　　　　　　表在性；（OIS Grade Ⅰ または Ⅱ）

544214.3　　　　　　　被膜下，表面積の50％を超える，非限局性；被膜下または実質内の損傷；
　　　　　　　　　　　実質内，直径5 cmを超える，非限局性；大；（OIS Grade Ⅲ）

544220.2　　　　　裂傷・裂創　詳細不明
544222.2　　　　　　　実質の深さ3 cm以下の単純な被膜裂傷；
　　　　　　　　　　　主要血管（脾柱）の損傷を伴わない；小；表在性；
　　　　　　　　　　　（OIS Grade Ⅰ または Ⅱ）

544224.3　　　　　　　脾門部損傷を伴わない部分的な実質損傷；
　　　　　　　　　　　深さ3 cmを超える，または主要血管（脾柱）の損傷；中（OIS Grade Ⅲ）

544226.4　　　　　　　脾門部離断を伴わないが脾臓の25％を超える血行遮断を生じるような実質損傷
　　　　　　　　　　　または脾門部血管の損傷；大（OIS Grade Ⅳ）

544228.5　　　　　　　完全な血行遮断を生じる脾門部離断；組織欠損；断裂；粉砕；広範囲；
　　　　　　　　　　　（OIS Grade Ⅴ）

ABDOMEN AND PELVIC CONTENTS

CODE	INJURY DESCRIPTION

	Spleen (continued)
544240.3	rupture ("fracture") NFS
	Use this code only when a more detailed description is not available.
544499.2	**Stomach** NFS
544410.2	contusion (hematoma) (OIS Grade I)
544420.2	laceration NFS
544422.2	no perforation; partial thickness (OIS Grade I)
544424.3	perforation; full thickness (OIS Grades II and III)
544426.4	avulsion; complex; rupture; tissue loss; with major vessel involvement; massive (OIS Grades IV and V)
544699.1	**Testes** NFS
544610.1	contusion (hematoma)
544620.1	laceration NFS
544622.1	minor, superficial
544624.2	avulsion; amputation; complex; rupture; massive
544899.2	**Ureter** NFS
544810.2	contusion (hematoma) (OIS Grade I)
544820.2	laceration NFS
544822.2	no perforation; partial thickness (OIS Grade II)
544824.3	perforation; full thickness (OIS Grade III)
544826.3	massive; avulsion; complex; rupture; tissue loss; transection (OIS Grades IV and V)
545099.2	**Urethra** NFS
545010.2	contusion (hematoma) (OIS Grade I)
545020.2	laceration NFS
545022.2	no perforation; partial thickness (OIS Grade III)
545024.3	perforation; full thickness (OIS Grade IV)
545026.3	avulsion; complex; rupture; tissue loss; massive (OIS Grade IV)
545028.4	with posterior tissue loss (OIS Grade V)
545299.1	**Uterus** NFS
545210.2	contusion (hematoma) (OIS Grade I)
545220.2	laceration (perforation) NFS
545222.2	≤1cm; minor; superficial (OIS Grade II)
545226.3	if pregnancy in 2nd trimester or 3rd trimester
545230.3	>1cm; placental abruption ≤50% major, deep (OIS Grade III)
545234.3	if pregnancy in 2nd trimester
545236.4	if pregnancy in 3rd trimester
545240.3	involving uterine artery; placental abruption >50%; massive; avulsion; complex; rupture (OIS Grades IV and V)
545242.4	if pregnancy in 2nd trimester
545246.5	if pregnancy in 3rd trimester

コード	損傷内容

脾臓（続き）

544240.3 　　　破裂（"fracture"） 詳細不明
　　　　　　　より詳細な情報のない場合のみこのコードを選択する。

544499.2 　胃　詳細不明
544410.2 　　　　挫傷（血腫）（OIS Grade Ⅰ）
544420.2 　　　　裂傷・裂創　詳細不明
544422.2 　　　　　　穿孔なし；非全層性（OIS Grade Ⅰ）
544424.3 　　　　　　穿孔あり；全層性（OIS Grade ⅡおよびⅢ）

544426.4 　　　　　　断裂；複雑；破裂；組織欠損；主要血管の損傷を伴う；広範囲
　　　　　　　　　　（OIS Grade ⅣおよびⅤ）

544699.1 　睾丸　詳細不明
544610.1 　　　　挫傷（血腫）
544620.1 　　　　裂傷・裂創　詳細不明
544622.1 　　　　　　小；表在性
544624.2 　　　　　　断裂；切断；複雑；破裂；広範囲

544899.2 　尿管　詳細不明
544810.2 　　　　挫傷（血腫）（OIS Grade Ⅰ）
544820.2 　　　　裂傷・裂創　詳細不明
544822.2 　　　　　　穿孔なし；非全層性（OIS Grade Ⅱ）
544824.3 　　　　　　穿孔あり；全層性（OIS Grade Ⅲ）
544826.3 　　　　　　広範囲；断裂；複雑；破裂；組織欠損；離断（OIS Grade ⅣおよびⅤ）

545099.2 　尿道　詳細不明
545010.2 　　　　挫傷（血腫）（OIS Grade Ⅰ）
545020.2 　　　　裂傷・裂創　詳細不明
545022.2 　　　　　　穿孔なし；非全層性（OIS Grade Ⅲ）
545024.3 　　　　　　穿孔あり；全層性（OIS Grade Ⅳ）
545026.3 　　　　　　断裂；複雑；破裂；組織欠損；広範囲（OIS Grade Ⅳ）
545028.4 　　　　　　　後部尿道組織の欠損を伴う（OIS Grade Ⅴ）

545299.1 　子宮　詳細不明
545210.2 　　　　挫傷（血腫）（OIS Grade Ⅰ）
545220.2 　　　　裂傷・裂創（穿孔）　詳細不明
545222.2 　　　　　　1 cm 以下；小；表在性（OIS Grade Ⅱ）
545226.3 　　　　　　　妊娠第2期（14週以降27週まで）または妊娠第3期（28週以降）
545230.3 　　　　　　1 cm 以上；50％以下の胎盤剥離；大；深在性（OIS Grade Ⅲ）
545234.3 　　　　　　　妊娠第2期
545236.4 　　　　　　　妊娠第3期
545240.3 　　　　　　子宮動脈の損傷を伴う；50％を超える胎盤剥離；広範囲；断裂；複雑；
　　　　　　　　　　　破裂（OIS Grade ⅣおよびⅤ）
545242.4 　　　　　　　妊娠第2期
545246.5 　　　　　　　妊娠第3期

CODE	INJURY DESCRIPTION
545499.1	**Vagina** NFS
545410.1	contusion (hematoma) (OIS Grade I)
545420.1	laceraiton (perforation) NFS
545422.1	minor; superficial (OIS Grade II)
545424.2	major; deep (OIS Grade III)
545426.3	massive; avulsion; complex; rupture (OIS Grade IV and V)
545699.1	**Vulva** NFS
545610.1	contusion (hematoma) (OIS Grade I)
545620.1	laceration (perforation) NFS
545622.1	minor, superficial (OIS Grade II)
545624.2	major, deep (OIS Grade III)
545626.3	massive; avulsion; complex; rupture (OIS Grade IV and V)

SKELETAL

Lumbar spine see SPINE

Pelvis see EXTREMITIES INCLUDING BONY PELVIS

Rib cage see THORAX

コード	損傷内容

545499.1　**腟**　詳細不明
545410.1　　　　挫傷（血腫）（OIS Grade Ⅰ）
545420.1　　　　裂傷・裂創（穿孔）　詳細不明
545422.1　　　　　　小；表在性（OIS Grade Ⅱ）
545424.2　　　　　　大；深在性（OIS Grade Ⅲ）
545426.3　　　　　　広範囲；断裂；複雑；破裂（OIS Grade ⅣおよびⅤ）

545699.1　**外陰部**　詳細不明
545610.1　　　　挫傷（血腫）（OIS Grade Ⅰ）
545620.1　　　　裂傷・裂創（穿孔）　詳細不明
545622.1　　　　　　小；表在性（OIS Grade Ⅱ）
545624.2　　　　　　大；深在性（OIS Grade Ⅲ）
545626.3　　　　　　広範囲；断裂；複雑；破裂（OIS Grade ⅣおよびⅤ）

骨　格

　　　腰椎　脊椎を参照

　　　骨盤　下肢を参照

　　　胸郭　胸部を参照

脊　椎

CERVICAL SPINE

CODE	INJURY DESCRIPTION

> Code paralysis according to its status at 24 hours post injury. If fatal, code status at time of death.

630299.2	**Brachial plexus** injury NFS [includes trunks, divisions or cords]
630210.2	incomplete plexus injury NFS
630212.2	contusion (stretch injury)
630214.2	laceration
630216.2	avulsion
630220.2	complete plexus injury NFS
630222.3	contusion (stretch injury)
630224.3	laceration
630226.3	avulsion
640200.3	**Cord** contusion NFS [includes the diagnosis of compression or epidural or subdural hemorrhage within spinal canal documented by imaging studies or autopsy]
640201.3	with transient neurological signs but NFS as to fracure/dislocation
640202.3	with no fracture or dislocation
640204.3	with fracture
640206.3	with dislocation
640208.3	with fracture and dislocation
640210.4	incomplete cord syndrome (preservation of some sensation or motor function; includes anterior cord, central cord, lateral cord (Brown-Sequard) syndromes) but NFS as to fracture/dislocation
640212.4	with no fracture of dislocation
640214.4	with fracture
640216.4	with dislocation
640218.4	with fracture and dislocation
640220.5	complete cord syndrome NFS (quadriplegia or paraplegia with no sensation)
640221.5	C-4 or lower but NFS as to fracture/dislocation, or NFS as to site
640222.5	with no fracture or dislocation
640224.5	with fracture
640226.5	with dislocation
640228.5	with fracture and dislocation
640229.6	C-3 or higher but NFS as to fracure/dislocation
640230.6	with no fracture or dislocation
640232.6	with fracture
640234.6	with dislocation
640236.6	with fracture and dislocation
640240.5	**Cord** laceration [includes transection and crush] NFS
640242.5	incomplete (preservation of some sensation or motor function) but NFS as to fracture/dislocation
640244.5	with no fracture or dislocation
640246.5	with fracture
640248.5	with dislocation
640250.5	with fracture and dislocation

頸　椎

コード	損傷内容

> 受傷後24時間の状態によって麻痺のコードを選択する。それ以前の死亡例は死亡時のコードを選択する。

コード	損傷内容
630299.2	**腕神経叢**　［神経幹，神経索および神経束を含む］　詳細不明
630210.2	不全型神経叢損傷　詳細不明
630212.2	挫傷（伸展損傷）
630214.2	裂傷・裂創
630216.2	引き抜き損傷
630220.2	完全型神経叢損傷　詳細不明
630222.3	挫傷（伸展損傷）
630224.3	裂傷・裂創
630226.3	引き抜き損傷
640200.3	**頸髄**挫傷　［画像診断法あるいは剖検により証明された脊柱管内の圧迫や硬膜外，硬膜下血腫の診断を含む］　詳細不明
640201.3	一過性の神経症状を伴う　骨折・脱臼については不明
640202.3	骨折と脱臼を伴わない
640204.3	骨折を伴う
640206.3	脱臼を伴う
640208.3	骨折と脱臼を伴う
640210.4	不全麻痺（何らかの知覚あるいは運動機能の残存；前脊髄症候群，中心性脊髄症候群，外側脊髄症候群〔Brown-Sequard 症候群〕を含む）　骨折・脱臼については不明
640212.4	骨折と脱臼を伴わない
640214.4	骨折を伴う
640216.4	脱臼を伴う
640218.4	骨折と脱臼を伴う
640220.5	完全麻痺（知覚機能の消失した四肢麻痺または対麻痺）　詳細不明
640221.5	第4頸髄以下だが，骨折・脱臼については不明，もしくは部位については不明
640222.5	骨折と脱臼を伴わない
640224.5	骨折を伴う
640226.5	脱臼を伴う
640228.5	骨折と脱臼を伴う
640229.6	第3頸髄以上だが，骨折・脱臼については不明
640230.6	骨折と脱臼を伴わない
640232.6	骨折を伴う
640234.6	脱臼を伴う
640236.6	骨折と脱臼を伴う
640240.5	**頸髄**裂傷・裂創　［離断と挫滅を含む］　詳細不明
640242.5	不全麻痺（何らかの知覚あるいは運動機能の残存）　骨折・脱臼については不明
640244.5	骨折と脱臼を伴わない
640246.5	骨折を伴う
640248.5	脱臼を伴う
640250.5	骨折と脱臼を伴う

脊椎

CERVICAL SPINE

CODE	INJURY DESCRIPTION

        Cord laceration (continued)
640260.5   complete cord syndrome NFS (quadriplegia or paraplegia with no sensation or motor function)
640261.5   C-4 or or lower but NFS as to fracture/dislocation
640262.5   with no frcture or dislocation
640264.5   with fracture
640266.5   with dislocation
640268.5   with fracture and dislocation
640269.6   C-3 or higher but NFS as to fracure/dislocation
640270.6   with no fracture or dislocation
640272.6   with fracture
640274.6   with dislocation
640276.6   with fracture and dislocation

650299.2   **Disc** injury NFS
650200.2   herniation NFS
650202.2   without nerve root damage (radiculopathy)
650203.3   with nerve root damage (radiculopathy) ; ruptured disc

650204.2   Dislocation (subluxation) without fracture, cord contusion or cord laceration NFS
        ⟨code as one injury and assign to the superior vertebra⟩

650206.3   **atlanto-axial (odontoid)**
650208.2   **atlanto-occipital**
650209.2   **facet** NFS
650210.2   unilateral
650212.3   bilateral

650216.2   Fracture without cord contusion or laceration with or without dislocaion NFS
        ⟨code each vertebra separately⟩

650218.2   **spinous process**
650220.2   **transverse process**
650222.3   **facet**
650224.3   **lamia**
650226.3   **pedicle**
650228.3   **odontoid (dens)**
650230.2   **vertebral body** NFS ⟨Use for "burst fracture"⟩

650232.2   minor compression ($\leq 20\%$ loss of anterior height)
650234.3   major compression ($> 20\%$ loss of height)

640284.1   **Interspinous ligament** laceration (disruption)

630260.2   **Nerve root,** single or multiple, NFS
630202.2   contusion (stretch injury)
630204.2   laceration NFS
630206.2   single
630208.3   multiple
630262.2   avulsion NFS
630264.2   single
630266.3   multiple

640278.1   Strain, acute with no fracture or dislocation

コード	損傷内容

頸髄裂傷・裂創（続き）

コード	内容
640260.5	完全麻痺（知覚運動機能の消失した四肢麻痺または対麻痺）　詳細不明
640261.5	第4頸髄以下では，骨折・脱臼については不明
640262.5	骨折と脱臼を伴わない
640264.5	骨折を伴う
640266.5	脱臼を伴う
640268.5	骨折と脱臼を伴う
640269.6	第3頸髄以上では，骨折・脱臼については不明
640270.6	骨折と脱臼を伴わない
640272.6	骨折を伴う
640274.6	脱臼を伴う
640276.6	骨折と脱臼を伴う
650299.2	**椎間板**損傷　詳細不明
650200.2	ヘルニア　詳細不明
650202.2	神経根損傷（神経根障害）を伴わない
650203.3	神経根損傷（神経根障害）を伴う；椎間板破裂
650204.2	頸椎脱臼（亜脱臼）（骨折，頸髄挫傷，頸髄裂傷を伴わない）　詳細不明

上位頸椎の損傷として1つだけコードを選択する。

コード	内容
650206.3	環軸関節（歯突起）
650208.2	環椎後頭骨関節
650209.2	椎間関節　詳細不明
650210.2	片側
650212.3	両側
650216.2	頸椎骨折（頸髄挫傷，頸髄裂傷を伴わないが脱臼の有無は問わない）　詳細不明

各椎骨ごとにコードを選択する。

コード	内容
650218.2	棘突起
650220.2	横突起
650222.3	関節突起
650224.3	椎弓
650226.3	椎弓根
650228.3	歯突起（軸椎）
650230.2	椎体　詳細不明　　"破裂骨折"に使用
650232.2	小（椎体前面高の減少が20%以下）
650234.3	大（椎体前面高の減少が20%を超える）
640284.1	**棘間靱帯**裂傷・裂創（断裂）
630260.2	**神経根**　単発あるいは多発　詳細不明
630202.2	挫傷（伸展損傷）
630204.2	裂傷・裂創　詳細不明
630206.2	単発
630208.3	多発
630262.2	引き抜き損傷　詳細不明
630264.2	単発
630266.3	多発
640278.1	捻挫（急性で骨折や脱臼を伴わない）

CODE	INJURY DESCRIPTION

WHOLE AREA

> Use one of the following two descriptors where such vague information is the only description available, These descriptors allow a means for identifying the occurrence of spinal injury, but they do not allow the calculation of an accurate ISS in these patients.

615099.9 **Blunt/traumatic cervical spine** injury NFS
615999.9 Died without further evaluation, no autopsy

頸　椎

コード	損傷内容

全　域

> 不確定な情報しか得られない場合には，以下の2つのコードのうちいずれかを選択する。ただしこれらのコードを選択した場合に ISS は計算してはならない。

615099.9　　**鈍的頸椎**損傷　詳細不明
615999.9　　　　　死亡（詳細な評価なし）；剖検なし

THORACIC SPINE

CODE	INJURY DESCRIPTION

> Code paralysis according to its status at 24 hours post injury. If fatal, code status at death.

640400.3	**Cord** contusion NFS [includes the diagnosis of compression or epidural or subdural hemorrhage within spinal canal documented by imaging studies or autopsy]
640401.3	with transient neurological signs (paresthesia) but NFS as to fracture/dislocation
640402.3	with no fracture or dislocation
640404.3	with fracture
640406.3	with dislocation
640408.3	with fracture and dislocation
640410.4	incomplete cord syndrome (preservation of some sensation or motor function; includes lateral cord (Brown-Sequard) syndrome) but NFS as to fracture/dislocation
640412.4	with no fracture or dislocation
640414.4	with fracture
640416.4	with dislocation
640418.4	with fracture and dislocation
640420.5	complete cord syndrome (paraplegia with no sensation) but NFS as to fracture/dislocation
640422.5	with no fracture or dislocation
640424.5	with fracture
640426.5	with dislocation
640428.5	with fracture and dislocation
640440.5	**Cord** laceration [includes transection and crush] NFS
640442.5	incomplete (preservation of some sensation or motor function) but NFS as to fracture/dislocation
640444.5	with no fracture or dislocation
640446.5	with fracture
640448.5	with dislocation
640450.5	with fracture and dislocation
640460.5	complete cord syndrome (paraplegia with no sensation or motor functions) but NFS as to fracture/dislocation
640462.5	with no fracture or dislocation
640464.5	with fracture
640466.5	with dislocation
640468.5	with fracture and dislocation

胸　椎

コード	損傷内容

受傷後24時間の状態によって麻痺のコードを選択する。それ以前の死亡例は死亡時のコードを選択する。

640400.3　**胸髄**挫傷　[画像診断法あるいは剖検により証明された脊柱管内の圧迫や硬膜外，硬膜下血腫の診断を含む]　詳細不明
640401.3　　　　一過性の神経症状（知覚異常）を伴うが骨折・脱臼については不明
640402.3　　　　　　骨折と脱臼を伴わない
640404.3　　　　　　骨折を伴う
640406.3　　　　　　脱臼を伴う
640408.3　　　　　　骨折と脱臼を伴う

640410.4　　　　不全麻痺（何らかの知覚あるいは運動機能の残存；外側脊髄〔Brown-Sequard〕症候群を含む）　骨折・脱臼については不明

640412.4　　　　　　骨折と脱臼を伴わない
640414.4　　　　　　骨折を伴う
640416.4　　　　　　脱臼を伴う
640418.4　　　　　　骨折と脱臼を伴う

640420.5　　　　完全麻痺（知覚機能障害を伴う対麻痺）　骨折・脱臼については不明

640422.5　　　　　　骨折と脱臼を伴わない
640424.5　　　　　　骨折を伴う
640426.5　　　　　　脱臼を伴う
640428.5　　　　　　骨折と脱臼を伴う

640440.5　**胸髄**裂傷・裂創　[離断と挫滅を含む]　詳細不明
640442.5　　　　不全麻痺（何らかの知覚あるいは運動機能の残存）　骨折・脱臼については不明

640444.5　　　　　　骨折と脱臼を伴わない
640446.5　　　　　　骨折を伴う
640448.5　　　　　　脱臼を伴う
640450.5　　　　　　骨折と脱臼を伴う

640460.5　　　　完全麻痺（知覚運動機能の消失した対麻痺）　骨折・脱臼については不明

640462.5　　　　　　骨折と脱臼を伴わない
640464.5　　　　　　骨折を伴う
640466.5　　　　　　脱臼を伴う
640468.5　　　　　　骨折と脱臼を伴う

脊椎

THORACIC SPINE

CODE	INJURY DESCRIPTION

650499.2   **Disc** injury NFS
650400.2   herniation NFS
650402.2   without nerve root damage (radiculopathy)
650403.3   with nerve root damage (radiculopathy) ; ruptured disc

650404.2   Dislocation (subluxation) without fracture, cord contusion or cord laceration NFS
                 code as one injury and assign to the superior vertebra
650409.2   **facet** NFS
650410.2   unilateral
650412.3   bilateral

650416.2   Fracture without cord contusion or laceration with or without dislocation NFS
                 code each vertebra separately
650418.2   **spinous process**
650420.2   **transverse process**
650422.3   **facet**
650424.3   **lamina**
650426.3   **pedicle**
650430.2   **vertebral body** NFS **Use for "burst" fracture**
650432.2   minor compression (≤20% loss of anterior height)
650434.3   major compression (>20% loss of height)

640484.1   **Interspinous ligament** laceration (disruption)

630499.2   **Nerve root**, single or multiple, NFS
630402.2   contusion (stretch injury)
630404.2   laceration NFS
630406.2   single
630408.3   multiple
630410.2   avulsion (rupture)
630412.2   single
630414.3   multiple

640478.1   Strain, acute with no fracture or dislocation

WHOLE AREA

> Use one of the following two descriptors when such vague information is the only description available. These descriptors allow a means for identifying the occurrence of spinal injury, but they do not allow the calculation of an accurate ISS in these patients.

616099.9   **Blunt/traumatic thoracic spine** injury NFS
616999.9   Died without further evaluation, on autopsy

コード	損傷内容
650499.2	**椎間板**損傷　詳細不明
650400.2	ヘルニア　詳細不明
650402.2	神経根損傷（神経根傷害）を伴わない
650403.3	神経根損傷（神経根傷害）を伴う；椎間板破裂
650404.2	胸椎脱臼（亜脱臼）（骨折，胸髄挫傷，胸髄裂傷を伴わない）　詳細不明
	上位胸椎の損傷として1つだけコードを選択する。
650409.2	椎間関節　詳細不明
650410.2	片側
650412.3	両側
650416.2	胸椎骨折（胸髄挫傷，胸髄裂傷を伴わないが脱臼の有無は問わない）　詳細不明
	各椎骨ごとにコードを選択する。
650418.2	棘突起
650420.2	横突起
650422.3	関節突起
650424.3	椎弓
650426.3	椎弓根部
650430.2	椎体　詳細不明　"破裂骨折"に使用
650432.2	小（椎体前面高の減少が20％以下）
650434.3	大（椎体前面高の減少が20％を超える）
640484.1	**棘間靱帯**裂傷・裂創（断裂）
630499.2	**神経根**　単発あるいは多発　詳細不明
630402.2	挫傷（伸展損傷）
630404.2	裂傷・裂創　詳細不明
630406.2	単発
630408.3	多発
630410.2	引き抜き損傷（断裂）
630412.2	単発
630414.3	多発
640478.1	捻挫（急性で骨折や脱臼を伴わない）

全　域

不確定な情報しか得られない場合には，以下の2つのコードのうちいずれかを選択する。ただしこれらのコードを選択した場合にISSは計算してはならない。

616099.9	**鈍的胸椎**損傷　詳細不明
616999.9	死亡（詳細な評価なし）；剖検なし

LUMBAR SPINE

CODE	INJURY DESCRIPTION

Code paralysis according to status hours post injury. If fatal, code status at death.

630600.3	**Cauda equina** contusion NFS
630602.3	with transient neurological signs (paresthesia) but NFS as to fracture/dislocation
630604.3	with no fracture or dislocation
630606.3	with fracture
630608.3	with dislocation
630610.3	with fracture and dislocation
630620.3	incomplete cauda equina syndrome but NFS as to fracture/dislocation
630622.3	with no fracture or dislocation
630624.3	with fracture
630626.3	with dislocation
630628.3	with fracture and dislocation
630630.4	complete cauda equina syndrome but NFS as to fracture/dislocation
630632.4	with no fracture or dislocation
630634.4	with fracture
630636.4	with dislocation
630638.4	with fracture and dislocation
640600.3	**Cord** contusion [includes the diagnosis of compression or epidural or subdural hemorrhage within spinal canal documented by imaging studies or autopsy] NFS
640601.3	with transient neurological signs but NFS as to fracture/dislocation
640602.3	with no fracture or dislocation
640604.3	with fracture
640606.3	with dislocation
640608.3	with fracture and dislocation
640610.4	incomplete cord syndrome (preservation of some sensation or motor function; includes lateral cord (Brown-Sequard syndrome) but NFS as to fracture/dislocation
640612.4	with no fracture or dislocation
640614.4	with fracture
640616.4	with dislocation
640618.4	with fracture and dislocation
640620.5	complete cord syndrome (paraplegia with no sensation or motor function) but NFS as to fracture/dislocation
640622.5	without fracture or dislocation
640624.5	with fracture
640626.5	with dislocation
640628.5	with fracture and dislocation
640640.5	**Cord** laceration [includes transection and crush] NFS
640642.5	incomplete (preservation of some sensation or motor function) but NFS as to fracture/dislocation
640644.5	with no fracture or dislocation
640646.5	with fracture
640648.5	with dislocation
640650.5	with fracture and dislocation
640660.5	complete cord syndrome (paraplegia with no sensation) but NFS as to fracture/dislocation
640662.5	with no fracture or dislocation
640664.5	with fracture
640666.5	with dislocation
640668.5	with fracture and dislocation

腰　椎

コード	損傷内容

受傷後24時間の状態によって麻痺のコードを選択する。それ以前の死亡例は死亡時のコードを選択する。

630600.3　**馬尾**挫傷
630602.3　　　　一過性の神経症状（知覚異常）を伴う　骨折・脱臼については不明
630604.3　　　　　　　　骨折と脱臼を伴わない
630606.3　　　　　　　　骨折を伴う
630608.3　　　　　　　　脱臼を伴う
630610.3　　　　　　　　骨折と脱臼を伴う
630620.3　　　　不全馬尾症候群　骨折・脱臼については不明
630622.3　　　　　　　　骨折と脱臼を伴わない
630624.3　　　　　　　　骨折を伴う
630626.3　　　　　　　　脱臼を伴う
630628.3　　　　　　　　骨折と脱臼を伴う
630630.4　　　　完全馬尾症候群　骨折・脱臼については不明
630632.4　　　　　　　　骨折と脱臼を伴わない
630634.4　　　　　　　　骨折を伴う
630636.4　　　　　　　　脱臼を伴う
630638.4　　　　　　　　骨折と脱臼を伴う

640600.3　**腰髄**挫傷　［画像診断法あるいは剖検により証明された脊柱管内の圧迫や硬膜外，硬膜下血腫の診断を含む］　詳細不明
640601.3　　　　一過性の神経症状を伴う　骨折・脱臼については不明
640602.3　　　　　　　　骨折と脱臼を伴わない
640604.3　　　　　　　　骨折を伴う
640606.3　　　　　　　　脱臼を伴う
640608.3　　　　　　　　骨折と脱臼を伴う

640610.4　　　　不全麻痺（何らかの知覚あるいは運動機能の残存；外側脊髄〔Brown-Sequard〕症候群を含む）骨折・脱臼については不明
640612.4　　　　　　　　骨折と脱臼を伴わない
640614.4　　　　　　　　骨折を伴う
640616.4　　　　　　　　脱臼を伴う
640618.4　　　　　　　　骨折と脱臼を伴う

640620.5　　　　完全麻痺（知覚運動機能の消失した対麻痺）　骨折・脱臼については不明
640622.5　　　　　　　　骨折と脱臼を伴わない
640624.5　　　　　　　　骨折を伴う
640626.5　　　　　　　　脱臼を伴う
640628.5　　　　　　　　骨折と脱臼を伴う

640640.5　**腰髄**裂傷・裂創　［離断と挫滅を含む］　詳細不明
640642.5　　　　不全麻痺（何らかの知覚あるいは運動機能の残存）　骨折・脱臼については不明
640644.5　　　　　　　　骨折と脱臼を伴わない
640646.5　　　　　　　　骨折を伴う
640648.5　　　　　　　　脱臼を伴う
640650.5　　　　　　　　骨折と脱臼を伴う

640660.5　　　　完全麻痺（知覚機能の消失した対麻痺）　骨折・脱臼については不明
640662.5　　　　　　　　骨折と脱臼を伴わない
640664.5　　　　　　　　骨折を伴う
640666.5　　　　　　　　脱臼を伴う
640668.5　　　　　　　　骨折と脱臼を伴う

脊椎

LUMBAR SPINE

CODE	INJURY DESCRIPTION
650699.2	**Disc** injury NFS
650600.2	herniation NFS
650602.2	without nerve root damage (radiculopathy)
650603.3	with nerve root damage (radiculopathy) ; ruptured disc
650604.2	**Dislocation** (subluxation) without fracture, cord contusion or cord laceration NFS
	code as one injury and assign to the superior vertebra
650609.2	**facet** NFS
650610.2	unilateral
650612.3	bilateral
650616.2	**Fracture** without cord contusion or laceration with or without dislocation NFS
	code each vertebra separately
650618.2	**spinous process**
650620.2	**transverse process**
650622.3	**facet**
650624.3	**lamina**
650626.3	**pedicle**
650630.2	**vertebral body** NFS
650632.2	minor compression ($\leq$20% loss of anterior height)
650634.3	major compression (>20% loss of height)
640684.1	**Interspinous ligament** laceration (disruption)
630699.2	**Nerve root or sacral plexus**, single or multiple, NFS
630660.2	contusion (stretch injury)
630662.2	laceration NFS
630664.2	single
630666.3	multiple
630668.2	avulsion (rupture) NFS
630612.2	single
630614.3	multiple
640678.1	Strain, acute with no fracture or dislocation

WHOLE AREA

Use one of the following two descriptors when vague information is the only description available. These descriptors allow a means for identifying the occurrence of spinal injury, but they do not allow the calculation of an accurate ISS in these patients.

617099.9	**Blunt/traumatic lumbar spine** injury NFS
617999.9	Died without further evaluation; no autopsy.

コード	損傷内容

- 650699.2　**椎間板**損傷　詳細不明
- 650600.2　　　ヘルニア　詳細不明
- 650602.2　　　　　神経根損傷（神経根傷害）を伴わない
- 650603.3　　　　　神経根損傷（神経根傷害）を伴う；椎間板破裂

- 650604.2　腰椎脱臼（亜脱臼）（骨折，腰髄挫傷，腰髄裂傷を伴わない）　詳細不明
  > 上位腰椎の損傷として1つだけコード選択する。
- 650609.2　　　**椎間関節**　詳細不明
- 650610.2　　　　　片側
- 650612.3　　　　　両側

- 650616.2　腰椎骨折（腰髄挫傷，腰髄裂傷を伴わないが脱臼の有無は問わない）　詳細不明
  > 各椎体ごとにコードを選択する。
- 650618.2　　　**棘突起**
- 650620.2　　　**横突起**
- 650622.3　　　**関節突起**
- 650624.3　　　**椎弓**
- 650626.3　　　**椎弓根部**
- 650630.2　　　**椎体**　詳細不明
- 650632.2　　　　　小（椎体前面高の減少が20％以下）
- 650634.3　　　　　大（椎体前面高の減少が20％を超える）

- 640684.1　**棘間靱帯**裂傷・裂創（断裂）

- 630699.2　**神経根あるいは仙骨神経叢**，単発あるいは多発　詳細不明
- 630660.2　　　挫傷（伸展損傷）
- 630662.2　　　裂傷・裂創　詳細不明
- 630664.2　　　　　単発
- 630666.3　　　　　多発
- 630668.2　　　引き抜き損傷（断裂）詳細不明
- 630612.2　　　　　単発
- 630614.3　　　　　多発

- 640678.1　捻挫（急性で骨折や脱臼を伴わない）

全域

> 不確定な情報しか得られない場合には，以下の2つのコードのうちいずれかを選択する。ただしこれらのコードを選択した場合にISSは計算してはならない。

- 617099.9　**鈍的腰椎**損傷　詳細不明
- 617999.9　　　死亡（詳細な評価なし）；剖検なし

上　肢

UPPER EXTREMITY

CODE	INJURY DESCRIPTION

WHOLE AREA

711000.3 **Amputation** (traumatic) at any point of extremity except finger

> see Skeletal-Bones for finger amputation

713000.3 Massive destruction of bone and of muscles/nervous system/vascular system of part or entire extremity (**Crush**)

Degloving injury
714002.2   arm or forearm
714004.2   finger (s) only, single or multiple
714006.3   hand, palm or entire extremity

715000.2 Extremity injury with compartment syndrome

> Use only if specific anatomical description is not available.

716000.1 **Penetrating injury** NFS

> Use only if more specific anatomic information is not available or if entire limb is involved. Penetrating injury through bone and tissue should be coded as open fracture to specific bone.

716002.1   superficial; minor
716004.2   with tissue loss $>25cm^2$
716006.3   with blood loss $>20\%$ by volume

> Assign one of the following codes, as appropriate, to soft tissue (external) injuries to the upper extremity. To calculate an ISS, however, assign these injuries to the External body region and follow rules for ISS calculation on pages xviii and xix.

710099.1 **Skin/Subcutaneous/muscle** NFS
710202.1   abrasion
710402.1   contusion (hematoma)
710600.1   laceration NFS
710602.1   minor; superficial

710604.2   major ($>$10cm long on hand or 20cm long on entire extremity and into sub-cutaneous tissue)

710606.3   blood loss $>20\%$ by volume
710800.1   avulsion NFS
710802.1   superficial; minor ($\leq 25cm^2$ on hand or $100cm^2$ on entire extremity)
710804.2   major ($>25cm^2$ on hand or $100cm^2$ on entire extremity)
710806.3   blood loss $>20\%$ by volume

上 肢

コード	損傷内容

全 域

711000.3　手指を除くすべての部位における（外傷性）**切断**

> 手指の切断については「骨格-骨－手指の切断」を参照

713000.3　上肢全体あるいは上肢の一部の，骨／筋肉／神経系／血管系の広範囲損傷（**挫滅**）

デグロービング損傷
714002.2　　　　上腕または前腕
714004.2　　　　手指のみ，単独または複数
714006.3　　　　手，手掌，あるいは上肢全体

715000.2　コンパートメント症候群を伴う上肢の損傷

> 他に明確な解剖学的情報がない場合にのみ使用する。

716000.1　**穿通性損傷**　詳細不明

> 他に明確な解剖学的情報がない場合あるいは上肢全体にわたる損傷の場合にのみ使用する。骨と組織を貫通する穿通性損傷は該当する骨の開放骨折としてコードを選択する。

716002.1　　　　表在性；小
716004.2　　　　$25cm^2$を超える組織欠損
716006.3　　　　出血量が全血液量の20％を超える

> 上肢の軟部組織（外表）損傷には，以下のコードの中で適切なものを選択する。ただしISSを算出する場合には，「上肢」ではなく「体表」の区分として取り扱い，21，22ページのISS計算ルールに従う。

710099.1　**皮膚／皮下／筋肉**　詳細不明
710202.1　　　　擦過傷
710402.1　　　　挫傷（血腫）
710600.1　　　　裂傷・裂創　詳細不明
710602.1　　　　　　小；表在性

710604.2　　　　　　大（手では10cm，手以外の上肢では20cmを超えかつ皮下組織に達する）

710606.3　　　　　　出血量が全血液量の20％を超える
710800.1　　　　剝離　詳細不明
710802.1　　　　　　表在性；小（手では$25cm^2$以下または上肢全体では$100cm^2$以下）
710804.2　　　　　　大（手では$25cm^2$または上肢全体では$100cm^2$を超える）
710806.3　　　　　　出血量が全血液量の20％を超える

UPPER EXTREMITY

CODE	INJURY DESCRIPTION

> Use one of the following two descriptors when such vague information is the only description available. These descriptors allow a means for identifying the occurrence of upper extremity injury, but they do not allow the calculation of an accurate ISS in these patients.

715099.9 **Blunt/traumatic upper extremity** injury NFS
715999.9   Died without further evaluation, no autopsy

VESSELS

> Vessel injuries are coded as separate injuries if: (1) they are isolated injuries (i. e., no accompanying documented organ injury) or (2) accompanying organ injury does not include any vessel injury description or (3) named vessel injury occurs with organ injury and is higher in severity than descriptor for organ injury.
> The terms "laceration," "puncture" and "perforation" are oftentimes used interchangeably to describe vessel injuries. When "puncture" or "perforation" is used, code as laceration. Descriptions for vessel lacerations distinguish between complete and incomplete transection. See footnotes "i" and "j".

720299.2 **Axillary artery** NFS
720202.2   intimal tear, no disruption
720204.2   laceration (perforation, puncture) NFS
720206.2   minor[i]
720208.3   major[j]

720499.2 **Axillary vein** NFS
720402.2   laceration (perforation, puncture) NFS
720404.2   minor[i]
720406.3   major[j]

720699.2 **Brachial artery** NFS
720602.2   intimal tear, no disruption
720604.2   laceration (puncture, perforation) NFS
720606.2   minor[i]
720608.3   major[j]

720899.1 **Brachial vein** NFS
720802.1   laceration (perforation, puncture) NFS
720804.1   minor[i] with or without thrombosis
720806.3   major[j]

721099.1 **Other named arteries** NFS (e. g., distal to elbow or small arteries of extremities)
721002.1   intimal tear, no disruption
721004.1   laceration (perforation, puncture) NFS
721006.1   minor[i]
721008.3   major[j]

---

[i] superficial; incomplete transection; incomplete circumferential involvement; blood loss ≤20% by volume
[j] rupture; complete transection; segmental loss; complete circumferential involvement; blood loss >20% by volume

コード	損傷内容

> 不確定な情報しか得られない場合には，以下の2つのコードのうちいずれかを選択する。ただしこれらのコードを選択した場合に ISS は計算してはならない。

715099.9　**上肢鈍的**損傷　詳細不明
715999.9　　　　死亡（詳細な評価なし）；剖検なし

血　管

> 血管損傷は，以下の場合には独立した損傷としてコードを選択する。
> (1)単独血管損傷（臓器損傷がない血管損傷）
> (2)臓器損傷に血管損傷に関する記載がないとき
> (3)血管損傷と臓器損傷が合併していて，血管損傷の重症度が臓器損傷の重症度より高いとき
> 血管損傷を表わす場合，"裂傷""穿刺""穿孔"などの用語はしばしば同じような意味で用いられる。血管の"穿孔"や"穿刺"と記載されている場合は"裂傷"としてコード選択する。血管の裂傷については，完全断裂と不全断裂に区分する。脚注 i, j を参照。

720299.2　**腋窩動脈**　詳細不明
720202.2　　　内膜剥離（断裂なし）
720204.2　　　裂傷・裂創（穿孔，穿刺）詳細不明
720206.2　　　　　小 [i]
720208.3　　　　　大 [j]

720499.2　**腋窩静脈**　詳細不明
720402.2　　　裂傷・裂創（穿孔，穿刺）詳細不明
720404.2　　　　　小 [i]
720406.3　　　　　大 [j]

720699.2　**上腕動脈**　詳細不明
720602.2　　　内膜剥離（断裂なし）
720604.2　　　裂傷・裂創（穿孔，穿刺）詳細不明
720606.2　　　　　小 [i]
720608.3　　　　　大 [j]

720899.1　**上腕静脈**　詳細不明
720802.1　　　裂傷・裂創（穿孔，穿刺）詳細不明
720804.1　　　　　小 [i]　血栓の有無を問わない
720806.3　　　　　大 [j]

721009.1　**その他の動脈**（例；肘部より末梢側の動脈や上肢の小動脈）　詳細不明
721002.1　　　内膜剥離（断裂なし）
721004.1　　　裂傷・裂創（穿孔，穿刺）詳細不明
721006.1　　　　　小 [i]
721008.3　　　　　大 [j]

---

[i] 表在性；不完全断裂；非全周性；出血量が全血液量の20%以下。
[j] 破裂；完全断裂；部分欠損；全周性；出血量が全血液量の20%を超える。

UPPER EXTREMITY

CODE	INJURY DESCRIPTION
721299.1	**Other named veins** NFS (e. g., distal to elbow or small veins of extremities)
721202.1	laceration NFS
721204.1	minor[i]
721206.3	major[j]

NERVES

Brachial plexus see Spine

730299.1	**Digital nerve** NFS
730202.1	contusion Use for diagnosis of "palsy"
730204.1	laceration

730499.1	**Median, radial, or ulnar nerve** NFS
730410.1	contusion Use this for diagnosis of "palsy"
730420.1	laceration NFS
730430.2	single nerve
730440.2	multiple nerves
730450.2	with motor loss

MUSCLES - TENDONS - LIGAMENTS

740200.1	**Tendon** laceration (rupture, tear, avulsion) NFS
740210.1	multiple tendons (in hand)
740220.1	multiple tendons (other than hand)
740400.2	**Muscle** laceration (rupture, tear, avulsion)
740402.1	strain, contusion
740600.2	**Joint capsule** laceration (rupture, tear, avulsion)

SKELETAL - JOINTS

750299.1	**Acromioclavicular joint** NFS
750210.1	contusion
750220.1	sprain
750230.2	dislocation (separation)
750240.2	laceration into joint

750499.1	**Carpal-Metacarpal or Metacarpal-Phalangeal joint,** including thumb NFS
750402.1	sprain
750404.1	dislocation

---

[i] superficial; incomplete transection; incomplete circumferential involvement; blood loss $\leq 20\%$ by volume
[j] rupture; complete transection; segmental loss; complete circumferential involvement; blood loss $>20\%$ by volume

コード	損傷内容
721299.1	その他の静脈（例；肘部より末梢側の静脈や上肢の小静脈）　詳細不明
721202.1	裂傷・裂創　詳細不明
721204.1	小 [i]
721206.3	大 [j]

神経

　　　腕神経叢　脊椎を参照

730299.1	指神経　詳細不明
730202.1	挫傷　"麻痺"の診断がある場合に使用
730204.1	裂傷・裂創
730499.1	正中神経，橈骨神経，尺骨神経　詳細不明
730410.1	挫傷　"麻痺"の診断がある場合に使用
730420.1	裂傷・裂創　詳細不明
730430.2	単一の神経
730440.2	複数の神経
730450.2	運動麻痺を伴う

筋肉ー腱ー靱帯

740200.1	腱裂傷・裂創（破裂，断裂，剥離）詳細不明
740210.1	複数（手）
740220.1	複数（手以外）
740400.2	筋肉裂傷・裂創（破裂，断裂，剥離）
740402.1	ストレイン（部分的過伸展損傷），挫傷
740600.2	関節包裂傷・裂創（破裂，断裂，剥離）

骨格ー関節

750299.1	肩鎖関節　詳細不明
750210.1	挫傷
750220.1	捻挫
750230.2	脱臼（離開）
750240.2	関節内に達する裂傷・裂創
750499.1	手根中手関節または中手指節関節，第一指を含む　詳細不明
750402.1	捻挫
750404.1	脱臼

---

[i] 表在性；不完全断裂；非全周性；出血量が全血液量の20％以下。
[j] 破裂；完全断裂；部分欠損；全周性；出血量が全血液量の20％を超える。

UPPER EXTREMITY

CODE	INJURY DESCRIPTION

750699.1 **Elbow joint** NFS
750610.1   contusion
750620.1   sprain
750630.1   dislocation with or without radial head involvement
750640.2   laceration into joint NFS
750642.2   with ligament involvement
750644.2   with single nerve laceration
750646.2   with multiple nerve lacerations
750650.3   massive destruction of bone and cartilage (crush)

750800.1 **Interphalangeal** dislocation

751099.1 **Shoulder (glenohumeral joint)** NFS
751010.1   contusion
751020.1   sprain
751030.2   dislocation
751040.2   laceration into joint
751050.3   massive destruction of bone and cartilage (crush)

751299.1 **Sternoclavicular joint** NFS
751210.1   contusion
751220.1   sprain
751230.2   dislocation
751240.2   laceration into joint

751499.1 **Wrist (carpus) joint** NFS
751410.1   contusion
751420.1   sprain
751430.2   dislocation at radiocarpal, intercarpal or pericarpal articulations
751440.2   laceration into joint
751450.3   massive destruction (crush) of bone and cartilage

SKELETAL - BONES

751600.2 **Acromion** fracture

751800.2 **Arm** fracture, NFS
> Use only if more specific anatomic information is unknown.

752000.2 **Carpus or Metacarpus** NFS
752002.2   fracture
752004.2   massive destruction (crush) of bone and cartilage

752200.2 **Clavicle** fracture (Grade I or II)

752400.1 **Finger** NFS
752402.2   amputation
752404.1   fracture
752406.2   massive destruction (crush) of bone and cartilage

コード	損傷内容

750699.1　肘関節　詳細不明
750610.1　　　　挫傷
750620.1　　　　捻挫
750630.1　　　　橈骨頭の脱臼の有無は問わない
750640.2　　　　関節内に達する裂傷・裂創　詳細不明
750642.2　　　　　　靭帯損傷を伴う
750644.2　　　　　　単独の神経裂傷・裂創を伴う
750646.2　　　　　　複数の神経裂傷・裂創を伴う
750650.3　　　　骨および軟骨の広範囲損傷（挫滅）

750800.1　指節間関節脱臼

751099.1　肩（肩関節）詳細不明
751010.1　　　　挫傷
751020.1　　　　捻挫
751030.2　　　　脱臼
751040.2　　　　関節内に達する裂傷・裂創
751050.3　　　　骨および軟骨の広範囲損傷（挫滅）

751299.1　胸鎖関節　詳細不明
751210.1　　　　挫傷
751220.1　　　　捻挫
751230.2　　　　脱臼
751240.2　　　　関節内の裂傷・裂創

751499.1　手関節　詳細不明
751410.1　　　　挫傷
751420.1　　　　捻挫
751430.2　　　　脱臼（橈骨手根関節，手根間関節または手根周囲の関節）
751440.2　　　　関節内に達する裂傷・裂創
751450.3　　　　骨および軟骨の広範囲損傷（挫滅）

骨格－骨

751600.2　肩峰骨折

751800.2　腕の骨折　詳細不明

> 他に明確な解剖学的情報がない場合にのみ使用する。

752000.2　手根骨または中手骨　詳細不明
752002.2　　　　骨折
752004.2　　　　骨および軟骨の広範囲損傷（挫滅）

752200.2　鎖骨骨折（GradeⅠまたはⅡ）

752400.1　手指　詳細不明
752402.2　　　　切断
752404.1　　　　骨折
752406.2　　　　骨および軟骨の広範囲損傷（挫滅）

UPPER EXTREMITY

CODE	INJURY DESCRIPTION
751900.2	**Forearm** fracture NFS
	Use only if more specific anatomic information is unknown.
752500.2	**Hand** fracture NFS
	Use only if more specific anatomic information is unknown.
752600.2	**Humerus** fracture NFS
752602.2	closed
752604.3	open/displaced comminuted any or combination
752606.3	with radial nerve involvement
752800.2	**Radius** fracture NFS with or without styloid process including Colles
752802.2	closed
752804.3	open/displaced/comminuted any or combination
752806.3	with radial nerve involvement
753000.2	**Scapula** fracture (OIS Grade II)
753200.2	**Ulna** fracture NFS
753202.2	closed
753204.3	open/displaced/comminuted any or combination
753206.3	with ulnar nerve involvement

コード	損傷内容

751900.2　前腕の骨折　詳細不明
　　　　　　他に明確な解剖学的情報がない場合にのみ使用する。

752500.2　手の骨折
　　　　　　他に明確な解剖学的情報がない場合にのみ使用する。

752600.2　上腕骨骨折　詳細不明
752602.2　　　　非開放
752604.3　　　　開放／転位／粉砕　いずれか1つ以上
752606.3　　　　橈骨神経の損傷を伴う

752800.2　橈骨骨折　詳細不明　茎状突起損傷（Colles骨折を含む）の有無を問わない
752802.2　　　　非開放
752804.3　　　　開放／転位／粉砕　いずれか1つ以上
752806.3　　　　橈骨神経の損傷を伴う

753000.2　肩甲骨骨折（OIS Grade Ⅱ）

753200.2　尺骨骨折　詳細不明
753202.2　　　　非開放
753204.3　　　　開放／転位／粉砕　いずれか1つ以上
753206.3　　　　尺骨神経の損傷を伴う

下　肢

LOWER EXTREMITY

CODE	INJURY DESCRIPTION

WHOLE AREA

811000.3 **Amputation** (traumatic) partial or complete but NFS as to site
811002.3   below knee; entire foot; calcaneus
811004.4   above knee

813000.2 Massive destruction of bone and of muscles/
nervous system/vascular system (**Crush**) but NFS as to site
813002.2   below knee, entire foot, calcaneus
813004.3   knee at or above

Degloving injury
814002.2   toe (s) only, single or multiple
814004.2   thigh, calf
814006.3   knee, ankle, sole of foot or entire extremity

815000.2 Extremity injury with compartment syndrome

> Use only if specific anatomic description is not available.

816000.1 **Penetrating injury** NFS

> Use only if more specific anatomic information is not available or if entire limb is involved. Penetrating injury to bone and tissue should be coded as open fracture to specific bone.

816002.1   superficial; minor
816004.2   with tissue loss >25cm^2
816006.3   with blood loss >20% by volume

> Assign one of the following codes, as appropriate, to soft tissue (external) injuries to the lower extremity. To calculate an ISS, however, assign these injuries to the External body region and follow rules for ISS calculation on pages xviii and xix.

810099.1 **Skin/Subcutaneous/muscle** NFS
810202.1   abrasion
810402.1   contusion (hematoma)
810600.1   laceration NFS
810602.1   minor, superficial
810604.2   major (>20cm long and into subcutaneous tissue)
810606.3   blood loss >20% by volume
810800.1   avulsion NFS
810802.1   superficial; minor; (≤100cm^2)
810804.2   major (>100cm^2)
810806.3   blood loss >20% by volume

下 肢

コード	損傷内容

全 域

811000.3　不全または完全**切断**　ただし切断の高さについては不明
811002.3　　　　　膝下；足部；踵部
811004.4　　　　　膝上

813000.2　骨格および筋肉／神経系／血管系の広範囲損傷（**挫滅**）　部位については不明

813002.2　　　　　膝下，足部，踵部
813004.3　　　　　膝または膝上

　　　　　デグロービング損傷
814002.2　　　　　足趾のみ，一趾あるいは複数趾
814004.2　　　　　大腿，腓腹部
814006.3　　　　　膝，足関節，足底，下肢全体

815000.2　コンパートメント症候群を伴う下肢の損傷

> 他に明確な解剖学的情報がない場合にのみ使用する。

816000.1　**穿通性損傷**　詳細不明

> 他に明確な解剖学的情報がない場合あるいは下肢全体にわたる損傷の場合にのみ使用する。骨と組織を貫通する穿通性損傷は該当する骨の開放骨折としてコードを選択する。

816002.1　　　　　表在性；小
816004.2　　　　　25cm^{2}を超える組織欠損
816006.3　　　　　出血量が全血液量の20%を超える

> 下肢の軟部組織（外表）損傷には，以下のコードの中で適切なものを選択する。ただしISSを算出する場合には，「下肢」ではなく「体表」の区分として取り扱い，21, 22ページのISS計算ルールに従う。

810099.1　**皮膚／皮下／筋肉**　詳細不明
810202.1　　　　　擦過傷
810402.1　　　　　挫傷（血腫）
810600.1　　　　　裂傷・裂創　詳細不明
810602.1　　　　　　小；表在性
810604.2　　　　　　大（長さ20cmを超え，かつ皮下組織に達する）
810606.3　　　　　　出血量が全血液量の20%を超える
810800.1　　　　　剝離　詳細不明
810802.1　　　　　　表在性；小（100cm^{2}以下）
810804.2　　　　　　大（100cm^{2}を超える）
810806.3　　　　　　出血量が全血液量の20%を超える

LOWER EXTREMITY

CODE	INJURY DESCRIPTION

> Use one of the following two descriptors when such vague information is the only description available. These descriptors allow a means for identifying the occurrence of lower extremity injury, but they do not allow the calculation of an accurate ISS in these patients.

815099.9 **Traumatic lower extremity** injury NFS
815999.9   Died without further evaluation; no autopsy

VESSELS

> Vessel injuries are coded as separate injuries if: (1) they are isolated injuries (i. e., no accompanying documented organ injury) or (2) accompanying organ injury does not include any vessel injury description or (3) named vessel injury occurs with organ injury and is higher in severity than descriptor for organ injury.
> The terms "laceration,""puncture" and "perforation" are oftentimes used interchangeably to describe vessel injuries. When "perforation" or "puncture" is used, code as laceration. Descriptions for vessel lacerations distinguish between complete and incomplete transection. See footnotes "i" and "j".

820299.3 **Femoral artery** NFS
820202.3   intimal tear, no disruption
820204.3   laceration (perforation, puncture) NFS
820206.3   minor[i]
820208.4   major[j]

820499.2 **Femoral vein** NFS
820402.2   laceration (perforation, puncture) NFS
820404.2   minor[i]
820406.3   major[j]

820699.2 **Popliteal artery** NFS
820602.2   intimal tear, no disruption
820604.2   laceration (perforation, puncture) NFS
820606.2   minor[i]
820608.3   major[j]

820899.2 **Popliteal vein** NFS
820802.2   laceration (perforation, puncture) NFS
820804.2   minor[i]
820806.3   minor[j]

821099.1 **Other named arteries** NFS (e. g., distal to knee or small lower extremity arteries)
821002.1   intimal tear, no disruption
821004.1   laceration (perforation, puncture) NFS
821006.1   minor[i]
821008.3   major[j]

---

[i] superficial; incomplete transection; incomplete circumferential involvement; blood loss ≤20% by volume
[j] rupture; complete transection; segmental loss; complete circumferential involvement; blood loss >20% by volume

コード	損傷内容

> 不確定な情報しか得られない場合には，以下の2つのコードのうちいずれかを選択する。ただしこれらのコードを選択した場合にはISSは計算してはならない。

815099.9　**下肢鈍的**損傷　詳細不明
815999.9　　　　　死亡（詳細な評価なし）；剖検なし

血 管

> 血管損傷は，以下の場合には独立した損傷としてコードを選択する。
> (1)単独血管損傷（臓器損傷がない血管損傷）
> (2)臓器損傷に血管損傷に関する記載がないとき
> (3)血管損傷と臓器損傷が合併していて，血管損傷の重症度が臓器損傷の重症度より高いとき
> 血管損傷を表わす場合"裂傷""穿刺""穿孔"などの用語はしばしば同じような意味で用いられる。血管の"穿孔"や"穿刺"と記載されている場合は"裂傷"としてコード選択する。血管の裂傷については，完全断裂と不全断裂に区分する。脚注 i，j を参照。

820299.3　**大腿動脈**　詳細不明
820202.3　　　　　内膜剥離（断裂なし）
820204.3　　　　　裂傷・裂創（穿孔，穿刺）　詳細不明
820206.3　　　　　　　　小[i]
820208.4　　　　　　　　大[j]

820499.2　**大腿静脈**　詳細不明
820402.2　　　　　裂傷・裂創（穿孔，穿刺）　詳細不明
820404.2　　　　　　　　小[i]
820406.3　　　　　　　　大[j]

820699.2　**膝窩動脈**　詳細不明
820602.2　　　　　内膜剥離（断裂なし）
820604.2　　　　　裂傷・裂創（穿孔，穿刺）　詳細不明
820606.2　　　　　　　　小[i]
820608.3　　　　　　　　大[j]

820899.2　**膝窩静脈**　詳細不明
820802.2　　　　　裂傷・裂創（穿孔，穿刺）　詳細不明
820804.2　　　　　　　　小[i]
820806.3　　　　　　　　大[j]

821099.1　**その他の動脈**（例；膝部より末梢の動脈や下肢の小動脈）　詳細不明
821002.1　　　　　内膜剥離（断裂なし）
821004.1　　　　　裂傷・裂創（穿孔，穿刺）　詳細不明
821006.1　　　　　　　　小[i]
821008.3　　　　　　　　大[j]

---

[i] 表在性；不完全断裂；非全周性；出血量が全血液量の20%以下。
[j] 破裂；完全断裂；部分欠損；全周性；出血量が全血液量の20%を超える。

LOWER EXTREMITY

CODE	INJURY DESCRIPTION

821299.1　**Other named veins** (e. g., distal to knee or small lower extremity veins) NFS
821202.1　　　laceration (perforation, puncture) NFS
821204.1　　　　　minor[i]
821206.3　　　　　major[j]

NERVES

830299.1　**Digital nerve** NFS
830202.1　　　contusion
830204.1　　　laceration

830499.2　**Sciatic nerve** NFS
830402.2　　　contusion (neurapraxia)
830404.3　　　laceration NFS
830406.3　　　　　incomplete
830408.3　　　　　complete

830699.2　**Femoral, tibial, peroneal nerve** NFS
830602.2　　　contusion
830604.2　　　laceration, avulsion NFS
830606.2　　　　　single nerve
830608.2　　　　　multiple nerves
830610.2　　　　　with motor loss

MUSCLE - TENDONS - LIGAMENTS

840200.2　**Achilles tendon** laceration (rupture, tear, avulsion) NFS
840202.2　　　incomplete
840204.2　　　complete

　　　　　Collateral or cruciate ligament laceration (rupture, tear, avulsion)
840402.2　　　ankle
840404.2　　　knee
840406.3　　　　　posterior cruciate with complete disruption

840600.2　**Muscle** laceration (rupture, tear, avulsion)
840602.1　　　strain, contusion

840802.2　**Tendon** laceration (rupture, tear, avulsion)
840804.2　　　multiple tendons

841002.2　**Patellar tendon** laceration (rupture, tear, avulsion)
841004.2　　　total transection

---

[i] superficial; incomplete transection; incomplete circumferential involvement; blood loss ≤20% by volume
[j] rupture; complete transection; segmental loss; complete circumferential involvement; blood loss >20% by volume

コード	損傷内容

821299.1　**その他の静脈**（例；膝部より末梢の静脈や下肢の小静脈）詳細不明
821202.1　　　　裂傷・裂創（穿孔，穿刺）詳細不明
821204.1　　　　小[i]
821206.3　　　　大[j]

神　経

830299.1　**趾神経**　詳細不明
830202.1　　　　挫傷
830204.1　　　　裂傷・裂創

830499.2　**坐骨神経**　詳細不明
830402.2　　　　挫傷（ニューラプラキシー）
830404.3　　　　裂傷・裂創　詳細不明
830406.3　　　　　　不完全
830408.3　　　　　　完全

830699.2　**大腿神経，脛骨神経，腓骨神経**　詳細不明
830602.2　　　　挫傷
830604.2　　　　裂傷・裂創，剥離　詳細不明
830606.2　　　　　　単一の神経
830608.2　　　　　　複数の神経
830610.2　　　　　　運動麻痺を伴う

筋肉―腱―靱帯

840200.2　**アキレス腱**裂傷・裂創（破裂，断裂，剥離）詳細不明
840202.2　　　　不完全
840204.2　　　　完全

　　　　　側副靱帯または十字靱帯の裂傷・裂創（破裂，断裂，剥離）
840402.2　　　　足関節部
840404.2　　　　膝部
840406.3　　　　　　後十字靱帯の完全断裂

840600.2　**筋肉**裂傷・裂創（破裂，断裂，剥離）
840602.1　　　　ストレイン（部分的過伸展損傷），挫傷

840802.2　**腱**裂傷・裂創（破裂，断裂，剥離）
840804.2　　　　多発性

841002.2　**膝蓋靱帯**裂傷・裂創（破裂，断裂，剥離）
841004.2　　　　完全断裂

---

[i] 表在性；不完全断裂；非全周性；出血量が全血液量の20%以下。
[j] 破裂；完全断裂；部分欠損；全周性；出血量が全血液量の20%を超える。

LOWER EXTREMITY

CODE	INJURY DESCRIPTION

SKELETAL - JOINTS

This section includes injuries that typically occur to joints (e. g., contusion, sprain, dislocation. It does not include fractures that occur to bones. These injuries are included under the section SKELETAL-BONES.

850299.1 **Ankle** NFS

Use only if specific anatomical information is unknown. If fibula, tibia or talus fracture is involved, code under specific bone. For lateral malleolus, see Fibula. For medial malleolus, see Tibia.

850202.1	contusion (involves articular cartilage)
850206.1	sprain
850210.2	dislocation NFS
850214.2	without involving articular cartilage
850218.2	involving articular cartilage
850222.2	laceration into joint

850400.1 **Foot joint** NFS Use this category only if specific anatomy is unknown.
850402.1   dislocation
850404.1   sprain

850699.1 **Hip** NFS For acetabulum, see Pelvis. For femoral head, see Femur.

850602.1	contusion (involves articular cartilage)
850606.1	sprain
850610.2	dislocation NFS
850614.2	without involving articular cartilage
850618.2	involving articular cartilage
850622.2	laceration into joint

850899.1 **Knee** NFS If femur, tibia, fibula or patella fracture is involved, code under specific bone.

850802.1	contusion (involves articular cartilage)
850806.2	dislocation NFS
850810.2	without involving articular cartilage
850814.2	involving articular cartilage
850818.2	laceration into joint
850822.2	meniscus tear
850826.2	sprain

851099.1 **Metatarsal, Phalangeal, or Interphalangeal joint** NFS
851002.1   sprain
851006.1   dislocation NFS
851010.1   without involving articular cartilage
851014.1   involving articular cartilage

851299.1 **Subtalar, transtarsal, or transmetatarsal joint** NFS
851202.1   sprain
851203.1   dislocation NFS
851204.1   without involving articular cartilage
851206.1   involving articular cartilage

コード	損傷内容

骨格一関節

> この章は関節に発生する典型的な損傷（例；挫傷，捻挫，脱臼）を含む。骨折は含まない。骨折については「骨格一骨」の章を参照。

850299.1　**足関節**　詳細不明
> 他に明確な解剖学的情報がない場合にのみ使用する。腓骨，脛骨，あるいは距骨の損傷を伴う場合は，それぞれの骨のコードに従う。外果については腓骨の項を参照。内果については脛骨の項を参照。

850202.1　　　　挫傷（関節軟骨の損傷を伴う）
850206.1　　　　捻挫
850210.2　　　　脱臼　詳細不明
850214.2　　　　　　　関節軟骨の損傷を伴わない
850218.2　　　　　　　関節軟骨の損傷を伴う
850222.2　　　　関節内裂傷・裂創

850400.1　**足部の関節**　詳細不明　　他に明確な解剖学的情報がない場合にのみ使用する。
850402.1　　　　脱臼
850404.1　　　　捻挫

850699.1　**股関節**　詳細不明　　寛骨臼については骨盤の項を参照。大腿骨頭については大腿骨の項を参照

850602.1　　　　挫傷（関節軟骨の損傷を伴う）
850606.1　　　　捻挫
850610.2　　　　脱臼　詳細不明
850614.2　　　　　　　関節軟骨の損傷を伴わない
850618.2　　　　　　　関節軟骨の損傷を伴う
850622.2　　　　関節内に達する裂傷・裂創

850899.1　**膝関節**　詳細不明
> 大腿骨，脛骨，腓骨あるいは膝蓋骨の損傷を伴う場合はそれぞれの骨のコードを選択する。

850802.1　　　　挫傷（関節軟骨の損傷を伴う）
850806.2　　　　脱臼　詳細不明
850810.2　　　　　　　関節軟骨の損傷を伴わない
850814.2　　　　　　　関節軟骨の損傷を伴う
850818.2　　　　関節内裂傷・裂創
850822.2　　　　半月板損傷
850826.2　　　　捻挫

851099.1　**中足趾節関節，趾節間関節**　詳細不明
851002.1　　　　捻挫
851006.1　　　　脱臼　詳細不明
851010.1　　　　　　　関節軟骨の損傷を伴わない
851014.1　　　　　　　関節軟骨の損傷を伴う

851299.1　**距骨下関節，足根間関節，足根中足関節**　詳細不明
851202.1　　　　捻挫
851203.1　　　　脱臼　詳細不明
851204.1　　　　　　　関節軟骨の損傷を伴わない
851206.1　　　　　　　関節軟骨の損傷を伴う

LOWER EXTREMITY

CODE	INJURY DESCRIPTION

SKELETAL - BONES

851400.2 **Calcaneus** fracture

851699.1 **Fibula** NFS
851602.1   contusion
851604.1   with peroneal nerve injury (palsy)
851605.2   fracture, any type but NFS as to site
851606.2   head, neck, shaft
851608.2   lateral malleolus
851610.2   open/displaced/comminuted `any or combination`
851612.2   bimalleolar or trimalleolar
851614.3   open/displaced/comminuted `any or combination`

851800.3 **Femur** fracture NFS as to site `If "hip fracture," see Pelvis`
851801.3   open/displaced/comminuted `any or combination`
851804.3   condylar
851808.3   head
851810.3   intertrochanteric
851812.3   neck
851814.3   shaft
851818.3   subtrochanteric
851822.3   supracondylar

852000.2 **Foot** fracture NFS `Use only if specific anatomic information is unknown.`

852002.2 **Leg** fracture NFS `only if specific anatomic information is unknown.`

852200.2 **Metatarsal or Tarsal** fracture

852400.2 **Patella** fracture

Pelvis
852600.2   fracture, with or without dislocation, of any one or combination; acetabulum, ilium, ischium, coccyx, sacrum, pubic ramus.

> Includes diagnosis of "hip fracture" if documented but not further described anatomically. Simple closed fractures of superior and inferior right or left rami are not coded as comminuted fractures, but as closed fracture.

852602.2   closed/undisplaced
852604.3   open/displaced/comminuted `any or combination`

852606.4   substantial deformation and displacement with associated vascular disruption or with major retroperitoneal hematoma; "open book" fracture. (NSF as to blood loss)
852608.4   blood loss ≤20% by volume
852610.5   blood loss >20% by volume

コード	損傷内容

骨格―骨

851400.2　踵骨骨折

851699.1　腓骨　詳細不明
851602.1　　　　挫傷
851604.1　　　　　　　腓骨神経損傷（麻痺）を伴う
851605.2　　　　骨折　詳細不明
851606.2　　　　　　　骨頭，頸部，骨幹部
851608.2　　　　　　　外果
851610.2　　　　　　　　　　開放／転位／粉砕　いずれか1つ以上
851612.2　　　　　　　両果，三果
851614.3　　　　　　　　　　開放／転位／粉砕　いずれか1つ以上

851800.3　大腿骨骨折　詳細不明　股関節骨折の場合は骨盤の項を参照
851801.3　　　　　　　　　開放／転位／粉砕　いずれか1つ以上
851804.3　　　　　　顆部
851808.3　　　　　　骨頭
851810.3　　　　　　転子間
851812.3　　　　　　頸部
851814.3　　　　　　骨幹部
851818.3　　　　　　転子下
851822.3　　　　　　顆上

852000.2　足部の骨折　詳細不明　他に明確な解剖学的情報がない場合にのみ使用する。

852002.2　脚（あし）の骨折　詳細不明　他に明確な解剖学的情報がない場合にのみ使用する。

852200.2　中足骨または足根骨骨折

852400.2　膝蓋骨骨折

　　　　　骨盤
852600.2　　　寛骨臼，腸骨，坐骨，尾骨，仙骨，恥骨枝の1箇所以上の骨折で脱臼の有無を問わない

> "股関節骨折"の診断が記載されているが，詳細不明の場合もこのコードを選択する。単純な左または右の恥骨上・下枝の骨折は，粉砕骨折ではなく非開放骨折としてコードを選択する。

852602.2　　　　　　　非開放／転位なし
852604.3　　　　　　　開放／転位／粉砕　いずれか1つ以上

852606.4　　　　　　　血管断裂または後腹膜大量血腫を伴う骨盤変形と変位；
　　　　　　　　　　　open book 骨折（出血量については不明）
852608.4　　　　　　　出血量が全血液量の20%以下
852610.5　　　　　　　出血量が全血液量の20%を超える

LOWER EXTREMITY

CODE	INJURY DESCRIPTION

852800.3   **Sacroilium** fracture with or without dislocation

853000.3   **Symphysis pubis** separation (fracture)

853200.2   **Talus** fracture

853499.1   **Tibia** NFS
853402.1   contusion
853404.2   fracture NFS, any type but NFS as to site
853405.3   open/displaced/comminuted any or combination
            bimalleolar [see 851612.2 and 851614.3]
853406.2   condyles (plateau)
853408.3   open/displaced/comminuted any or combination
853410.2   intercondyloid spine
853412.2   medial malleolus
853414.2   open/displaced/comminuted any or combination
853416.2   posterior malleolus
853418.3   open/displaced/comminuted any or combination
853420.2   shaft
853422.3   open/displaced/comminuted any combination
            trimalleolar [see 851612.2 and 851614.3]

853699.1   **Toe** NFS
853602.1   fracture
853604.2   amputation
853606.2   crush

コード	損傷内容
852800.3	**仙腸骨**骨折　脱臼の有無は問わない
853000.3	**恥骨結合**離開（骨折）
853200.2	**距骨**骨折
853499.1	**脛骨**　詳細不明
853402.1	挫傷
853404.2	骨折　詳細不明
853405.3	開放／転位／粉砕　いずれか1つ以上
	両果　[851612.2および851614.3参照]
853406.2	顆部（脛骨プラトー）
853408.3	開放／転位／粉砕　いずれか1つ以上
853410.2	顆間隆起
853412.2	内果
853414.2	開放／転位／粉砕　いずれか1つ以上
853416.2	後果
853418.3	開放／転位／粉砕　いずれか1つ以上
853420.2	骨幹部
853422.3	開放／転位／粉砕　いずれか1つ以上
	三果　[851612.2および851614.3参照]
853699.1	**足趾**　詳細不明
853602.1	骨折
853604.2	切断
853606.2	挫滅

体表
熱傷
他の外傷

EXTERNAL-Skin and Subcutaneous Tissue

CODE	INJURY DESCRIPTION

> This section should be used only if no information is available on a specific body part or area. Multiple minor external injuries to one or more body region should be coded as one injury (AIS 1) using this section, e. g., "overall abrasions"=910200.1 or "multiple lacerations"=910600.1.

910200.1   Abrasion

910400.1   Contusion (hematoma)

910600.1   Laceration

910800.2   Avulsion

914000.1   Degloving injury

916000.1   Penetrating injury

体表―皮膚および皮下組織

コード	損傷内容

この区分のコードは損傷の部位または範囲が示されていない場合に使用する。体の一部位または複数部位に軽い皮膚損傷が多数存在する場合はこの区分のコードを1つの損傷として選択してもよい。例；"全身擦過傷＝910200.1" "多発裂創＝910600.1"

910200.1 　　擦過傷

910400.1 　　挫傷（血腫）

910600.1 　　裂創

910800.2 　　剥離

914000.1 　　デグロービング損傷

916000.1 　　穿通性損傷

BURNS

CODE	INJURY DESCRIPTION

The following burn injury descriptions are not a substitute for a comprehensive burn scale, but only intended as gross estimates of the severity. Burns are assigned to the External body region for ISS. Total body surface (TBS) is assessed by using the diagram of "nines" that follows. For example, one entire upper extremity (all sides) is 9% of the TBS. When burns occur in varying degrees, use most serious burn.

Code	Degree	Total body Surface
912000.1	NFS	NFS
912002.1	1° >1 yr old	any
912003.1	1° ≤1 yr old	≤50%
912004.2	1° ≤1 yr old	>50%
912006.1	2°	<10%
912007.1	3°	≤100cm^2 (except face ≤25cm^2)
912008.2	3°	>100cm^2 (except face ≥25cm^2) up to 10%
912012.2	2° or 3° (or full thickness)	10-19%
912014.3	<5 years old	
912016.3	face/hand/genitalia involvement	
912018.3	2° or 3° (or full thickness)	20-29%
912020.4	<5 years old	
912022.4	face/hand/genitalia involvement	
912024.4	2° or 3° (or full thickness)	30-39%
912026.5	<5 years old	
912028.5	face/hand/genitalia involvement	
912030.5	2° or 3° (or full thickness)	40-89%
912032.6	2° or 3° including incineration	≥90%

If a burn amputation occurs at the time of the traumatic event (direct result), code as amputation in body region. Do not code burn separately. If amputation is required sometime after the event, the burn and not the amputation is coded. In this case, amputation would be considered treatment.

熱　傷

コード	損傷内容

以下の熱傷の記述は，重症度を大まかに評価したもので，広範囲熱傷の重症度スケールに代わるものではない。熱傷は ISS を計算するときは「体表」として計算する。以下に示すように，体表面積（TBS）は「9」の法則で評価する。例えば，一側の上肢（全面）の面積は 9％である。さまざまな深度の熱傷が混在する場合はもっとも深いものを選択する。

　　　　　　　　　熱傷深度　　　　　　　　　　　　　　　熱傷面積

912000.1　　詳細不明　　　　　　　　　　　　　　　詳細不明

912002.1　　Ⅰ度　1歳を超える　　　　　　　　　　熱傷面積を問わない

912003.1　　Ⅰ度　1歳以下　　　　　　　　　　　　50％以下

912004.2　　Ⅰ度　1歳以下　　　　　　　　　　　　50％を超える

912006.1　　Ⅱ度　　　　　　　　　　　　　　　　　10％未満
912007.1　　Ⅲ度　　　　　　　　　　　　　　　　　100cm^{2}以下（顔面の場合は25cm^{2}以下）
912008.2　　Ⅲ度　　　　　　　　　　　　　　　　　100cm^{2}を超え（顔面の場合は25cm^{2}以上），かつ10％未満

912012.2　　Ⅱ度またはⅢ度　　　　　　　　　　　　10〜19％
912014.3　　　　　5歳未満
912016.3　　　　　顔面／手／性器に及ぶ
912018.3　　Ⅱ度またはⅢ度　　　　　　　　　　　　20〜29％
912020.4　　　　　5歳未満
912022.4　　　　　顔面／手／性器に及ぶ
912024.4　　Ⅱ度またはⅢ度　　　　　　　　　　　　30〜39％
912026.5　　　　　5歳未満
912028.5　　　　　顔面／手／性器に及ぶ
912030.5　　Ⅱ度またはⅢ度　　　　　　　　　　　　40〜89％
912032.6　　Ⅱ度またはⅢ度　　　　　　　　　　　　90％以上
　　　　　　　　　炭化を含む

熱傷受傷時に熱傷による四肢の切断が発生した場合は，それぞれの区分の「切断」のコードを選択し，「熱傷」のコードを選択しない。熱傷受傷後に切断を要した場合は，切断ではなくて熱傷としてコードを選択する。この場合の切断は治療と考える。

BURNS

CODE	INJURY DESCRIPTION

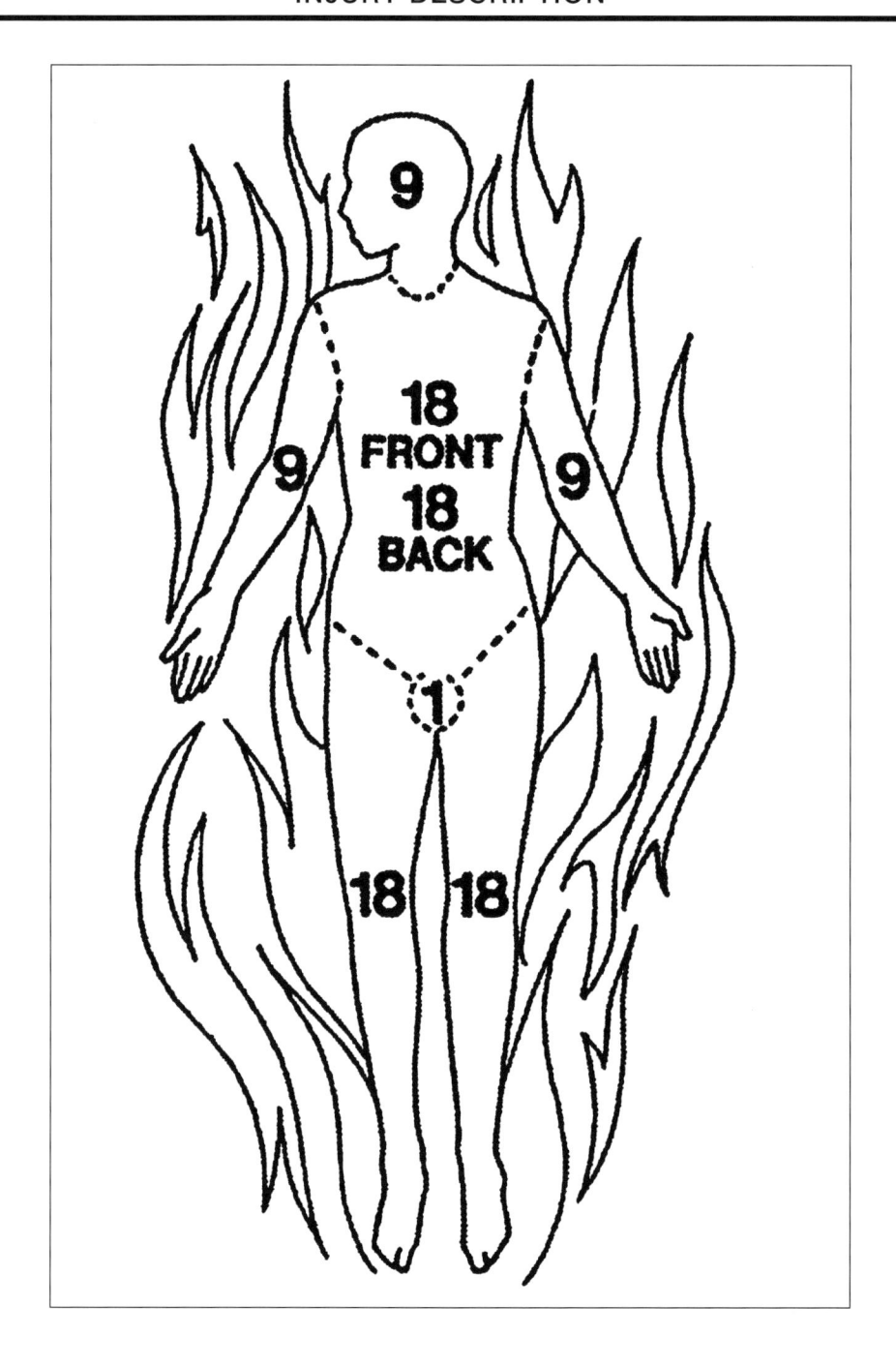

DIAGRAM OF NINES

Reprinted with permission of American Burn Association and American College of Surgeons.

コード	損傷内容

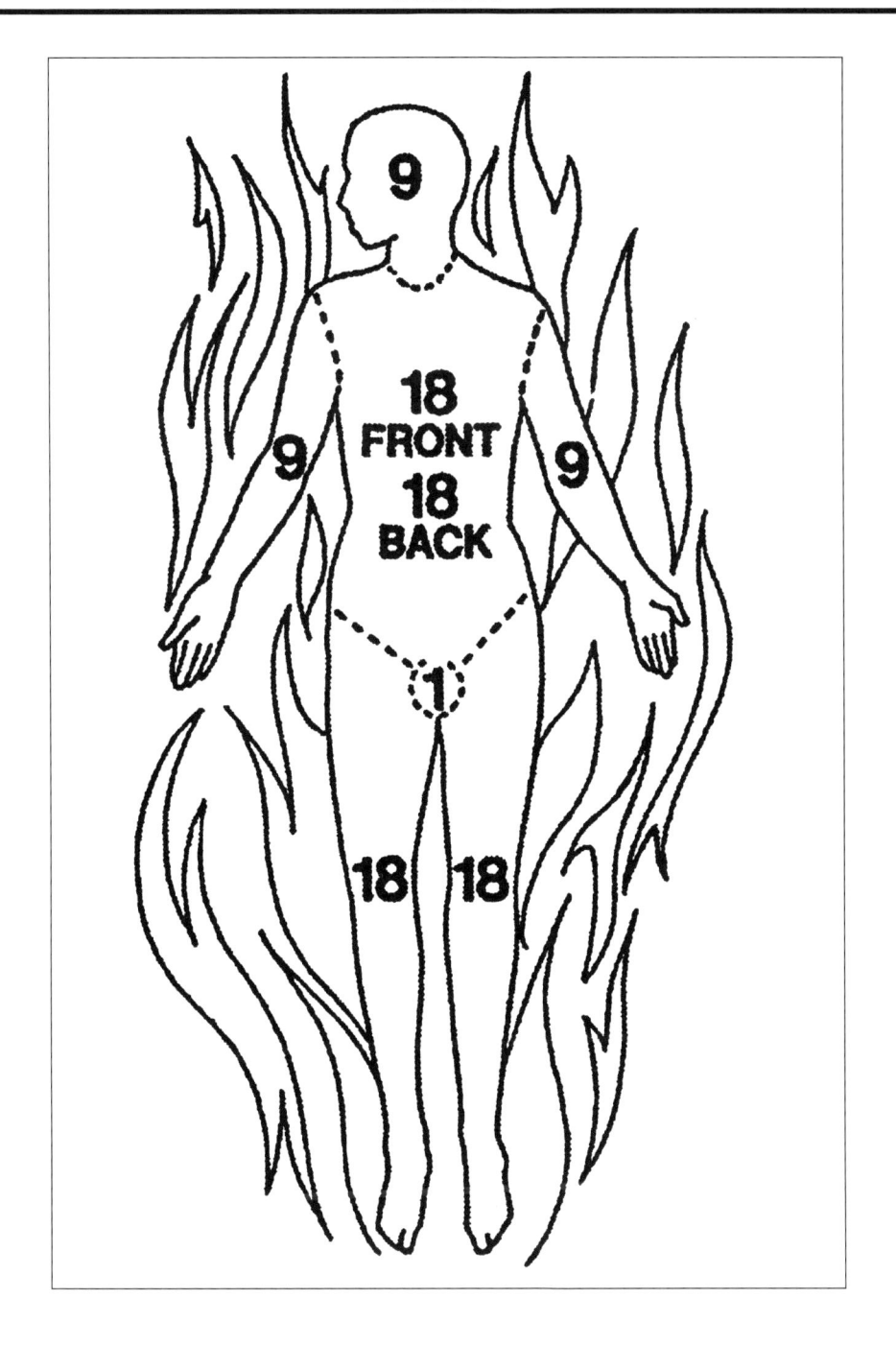

DIAGRAM OF NINES

米国外科学会および米国熱傷学会の許可を得て転載

OTHER TRAUMA

CODE	INJURY DESCRIPTION

919200.2   Inhalation injury NFS ⬚ Assign to THORAX region for ISS ⬚
919201.2   Absence of carbonaceous deposits, erythema, edema, bronchorrhea or obstruction

919202.3   Minor or patchy areas of erythema, carbonaceous deposits in proximal or distal bronchi ⬚ any or combination ⬚

919204.4   Moderate degree of erythema, carbonaceous deposits, bronchorrhea with or without compromise of the bronchi ⬚ any or combination ⬚

919206.5   Severe inflammation with friability, copious carbonaceous deposits, bronchorrhea, bronchial obstruction ⬚ any or combination ⬚

919208.6   Evidence of mucosal sloughing, necrosis, endoluminal obliteration ⬚ any or combination ⬚

919400.2   High voltage electrical injury ⬚ Assign to EXTERNAL region for ISS ⬚
919402.3   with muscle necrosis
919404.5   with cardiac arrest documented by medical personnel

他の外傷

コード	損傷内容

919200.2　吸入損傷(気道熱傷，腐食)　詳細不明　ISS を計算するときは「胸部」として扱う。
919201.2　　　以下の所見がない；すすの沈着，発赤，浮腫，気道分泌，気道閉塞

919202.3　　　軽度または斑状の発赤，近位または遠位の気管支へのすすの沈着
　　　　　　　いずれか1つ以上

919204.4　　　中等度の発赤，すすの沈着，気道分泌（ただし気管支傷害を問わない）
　　　　　　　いずれか1つ以上

919206.5　　　重度の炎症，多量のすすの沈着，多量の気道分泌，気管支閉塞
　　　　　　　いずれか1つ以上

919208.6　　　粘膜の脱落，壊死，内腔消失　いずれか1つ以上

919400.2　電撃傷　詳細不明　ISS を計算するときは「体表」として扱う。
919402.3　　　筋肉の壊死を伴う
919404.5　　　医療従事者により確認された心臓停止を伴う

DICTIONARY INDEX

Page	Anatomical Description	Section
46	Abdomen, whole area [use for Abdominal injury NFS, Penetrating or Skin]	Abdomen & Pelvic Contents
26	Abducens nerve	Head
71	Acetabulum [see Pelvis]	Lower Extremity
69	Achilles tendon	Lower Extremity
26	Acoustic nerve	Head
64	Acromioclavicular joint	Upper Extremity
65	Acromion	Upper Extremity
48	Adrenal gland	Abdomen & Pelvic Contents
34	Alveolar ridge [see also Teeth]	Face
70	Ankle	Lower Extremity
48	Anus	Abdomen & Pelvic Contents
	Aorta	
47	abdominal	Abdomen & Pelvic Contents
40	thoracic	Thorax
65	Arm NFS	Upper Extremity
26	Auditory nerve [see Acoustic nerve]	Head
63	Axillary artery	Upper Extremity
63	Axillary vein	Upper Extremity
24	Basilar artery	Head
48	Bladder (urinary)	Abdomen & Pelvic Contents
63	Brachial artery	Upper Extremity
55	Brachial plexus	Spine
63	Brachial vein	Upper Extremity
40	Brachiocephalic artery	Thorax
40	Brachiocephalic vein	Thorax
27	Brain stem	Head
39	Breast	Thorax
	Bronchus	
41	distal to main stem	Thorax
44	main stem	Thorax
71	Calcaneus	Lower Extremity
34	Canaliculus (tear duct)	Face
	Carotid artery	
37	common	Neck
33	external	Face
37	external	Neck
24	internal	Head
37	internal	Neck
24	Carotid - cavernous sinus	Head
64	Carpal joint [see Wrist, page 65]	Upper Extremity
64	Carpal - metacarpal joint	Upper Extremity
65	Carpus	Upper Extremity
60	Cauda equina	Spine
24	Cavernous sinus	Head
47	Celiac artery	Abdomen & Pelvic Contents
27	Cerebellum	Head

Page	Anatomical Description	Section
	Cerebral artery	
24	anterior	Head
24	middle	Head
25	posterior	Head
28	Cerebrum	Head
	Chest [see Thorax]	
42	Chordae tendinae	Thorax
34	Choroid	Face
65	Clavicle	Upper Extremity
71	Coccyx [see Pelvis]	Lower Extremity
69	Collateral ligament	Lower Extremity
48	Colon (large bowel)	Abdomen & Pelvic Contents
34	Conjunctiva	Face
34	Cornea	Face
40	Coronary artery	Thorax
25	Cranial nerve	Head
38	Cricoid cartilage [see Larynx]	Neck
69	Cruciate ligament [see Collateral ligament]	Lower Extremity
49	Cystic duct	Abdomen & Pelvic Contents
36	Decapitation	Neck
42	Diaphragm	Thorax
64	Digital nerve	Upper Extremity
69	Digital nerve	Lower Extremity
	Disc	
56	cervical	Spine
61	lumbar	Spine
59	thoracic	Spine
49	Duodenum	Abdomen & Pelvic Contents
34	Ear	Face
65	Elbow joint	Upper Extremity
42	Esophagus	Thorax
30	Ethmoid bone [see Skull, base]	Head
34	Eye	Face
33	Face, whole area [use for Penetrating or Skin]	Face
34	Facial bone (s) NFS	Face
26	Facial nerve	Head
51	Fallopian tube [see Ovarian tube]	Abdomen & Pelvic Contents
68	Femoral artery	Lower Extremity
69	Femoral nerve	Lower Extremity
68	Femoral vein	Lower Extremity
71	Femur	Lower Extremity
71	Fibula	Lower Extremity
65	Finger	Upper Extremity
	Foot	
70	joint NFS	Lower Extremity
71	bone NFS	Lower Extremity
66	Forearm NFS	Upper Extremity

Page	Anatomical Description	Section
30	Frontal bone [see Skull, vault]	Head
49	Gallbladder	Abdomen & Pelvic Contents
34	Gingiva (gum)	Face
65	Glenohumeral joint [see Shoulder, page 65]	Upper Extremity
26	Glossopharyngeal nerve	Head
66	Hand NFS	Upper Extremity
23	Head, whole area [use for Penetrating, Scalp, Head/Brain injury NFS, Crush]	Head
42	Heart	Thorax
70	Hip	Lower Extremity
66	Humerus	Upper Extremity
38	Hyoid bone	Neck
26	Hypoglossal nerve	Head
27	Hypothalamus [see Brain stem]	Head
49	Ileum (small bowel) [see Jejunum]	Abdomen & Pelvic Contents
47	Iliac artery (common, internal, external)	Abdomen & Pelvic Contents
47	Iliac vein (common, internal, external)	Abdomen & Pelvic Contents
71	Ilium [see Pelvis]	Lower Extremity
34	Inner ear	Face
40	Innominate artery [see Brachiocephalic artery]	Thorax
40	Innominate vein [see Brachiocephalic vein]	Thorax
65	Interphalangeal joint	Upper Extremity
70	Interphalangeal joint [see Metatarsal, Phalangeal or Interphalangeal joint]	Lower Extremity
42	Interventricular septum	Thorax
42	Inter-atrial septum [see interventricular septum]	Thorax
42	Intracardiac valve	Thorax
24	Intracranial vessel	Head
34	Iris	Face
71	Ischium [see Pelvis]	Lower Extremity
49	Jejunum (small bowel)	Abdomen & Pelvic Contents
64	Joint capsule NFS	Upeer Extremity
	Jugular vein	
37	external	Neck
37	internal	Neck
49	Kidney	Abdomen & Pelvic Contents
70	Knee	Lower Extremity
48	Large bowel [see Colon]	Abdomen & Pelvic Contents
38	Larynx	Neck
71	Lateral malleolus [see Fibula]	Lower Extremity
50	Liver	Abdomen & Pelvic Contents
67	Lower extremity, whole area [use for Penetrating, Skin, Degloving, Amputation, Crush, Compartment Syndrome]	Lower Extremity
42	Lung	Thorax
44	Main stem bronchus [see Trachea]	Thorax
35	Mandible	Face

79

Page	Anatomical Description	Section
35	Maxilla	Face
35	Maxillary sinus [see Maxilla]	Face
64	Median nerve	Upper Extremity
27	Medulla [see Brain stem]	Head
51	Mesentery	Abdomen & Pelvic Contents
64	Metacarpal - phalangeal joint [see Carpal-Metacarpal]	Upper Extremity
65	Metacarpus [see Carpus, page 65]	Upper Extremity
	Metatarsus	
70	joint	Lower Extremity
71	bone	Lower Extremity
27	Midbrain [see Brain stem]	Head
34	Middle ear [see Inner ear]	Face
34	Mouth	Face
64	Muscle NFS	Upper Extremity
69	Muscle NFS	Lower Extremity
42	Myocardium [see Heart]	Thorax
36	Neck, whole area [use for Penetrating or Skin]	Neck
	Nerve root	
56	cervical	Spine
61	lumbar	Spine
59	thoracic	Spine
35	Nose	Face
30	Occipital bone [see Skull, base or vault]	Head
26	Oculomotor nerve	Head
25	Olfactory nerve	Head
51	Omentum	Abdomen & Pelvic Contents
	Optic nerve	
26	intracranial segment	Head
26	intracananicular segment	Head
33	intraorbital segment	Face
35	Orbit [see also Optic nerve, intraorbital segment in Face, page 33]	Face
30	Orbital roof [see Skull, base]	Head
34	Ossicular chain (ear bone)	Face
51	Ovarian tube	Abdomen & Pelvic Contents
51	Ovary	Abdomen & Pelvic Contents
51	Pancreas	Abdomen & Pelvic Contents
30	Parietal bone [see Skull, vault]	Head
71	Patella	Lower Extremity
69	Patellar tendon	Lower Extremity
71	Pelvis	Lower Extremity
51	Penis	Abdomen & Pelvic Contents
43	Pericardium	Thorax
51	Perineum	Abdomen & Pelvic Contents
69	Peroneal nerve [see Femoral, tibial, peroneal nerve]	Lower Extremity

Page	Anatomical Description	Section
70	Phalangeal joint [see Metatarsal, Phalangeal or Interphalangeal joint]	Lower Extremity
38	Pharynx	Neck
38	Phrenic nerve	Neck
29	Pituitary gland	Head
52	Placenta	Abdomen & Pelvic Contents
43	Pleura	Thorax
27	Pons [see Brain stem]	Head
68	Popliteal artery	Lower Extremity
68	Popliteal vein	Lower Extremity
71	Pubic ramus	Lower Extremity
40	Pulmonary artery	Thorax
43	Pulmonary region [see Lung]	Thorax
40	Pulmonary vein	Thorax
64	Radial nerve [see Median, radial or ulnar nerve]	Upper Extremity
66	Radius	Upper Extremity
52	Rectum	Abdomen & Pelvic Contents
34	Retina	Face
52	Retroperitoneum	Abdomen & Pelvic Contents
38	Retropharyngeal area [see Pharynx]	Neck
45	Rib cage	Thorax
61	Sacral plexus [see Nerve root, page 61]	Spine
72	Sacroilium	Lower Extremity
71	Sacrum [see Pelvis]	Lower Extremity
25	Saggital sinus [see Superior longitudinal sinus]	Head
38	Salivary gland	Neck
23	Scalp	Head
66	Scapula	Upper Extremity
69	Sciatic nerve	Lower Extremity
34	Sclera	Face
52	Scrotum	Abdomen & Pelvic Contents
65	Shoulder	Upper Extremity
25	Sigmoid sinus	Head
25	Sinus	Head
	Skull	
30	base	Head
30	vault	Head
30	Sphenoid bone [see Skull, base or vault]	Head
26	Spinal accessory nerve	Head
	Spinal cord	
55	cervical	Spine
60	lumbar	Spine
58	thoracic	Spine
52	Spleen	Abdomen & Pelvic Contents
65	Sternoclavicular joint	Upper Extremity
45	Sternum	Thorax
53	Stomach	Abdomen & Pelvic Contents

Page	Anatomical Description	Section
40	Subclavian artery	Thorax
41	Suclavian vein	Thorax
70	Subtalar joint	Lower Extremity
25	Superior longitudinal sinus	Head
72	Symphysis pubis	Lower Extremity
72	Talus	Lower Extremity
71	Tarsus [see Metatarsal of Tarsal]	Lower Extremity
35	Teeth [see also Alveolar ridge in Face, page 34]	Face
30	Temporal bone [see Skull, base or vault]	Head
35	Temporomandibular joint	Face
64	Tendon NFS	Upper Extremity
69	Tendon NFS	Lower Extremity
53	Testes	Abdomen & Pelvic Contents
43	Thoracic cavity [see also Thorax, whole area, page 39]	Thorax
44	Thoracic duct	Thorax
39	Thorax, whole area [use for chest injury NFS, Penetrating or Skin; see also Thoracic cavity, page 43]	Thorax
38	Thyroid cartilage [see Larynx]	Neck
38	Thyroid gland	Neck
72	Tibia	Lower Extremity
69	Tibial nerve [see Femoral, tibial, peroneal nerve]	Lower Extremity
72	Toe	Lower Extremity
34	Tongue	Face
44	Trachea	Thorax
70	Transmetatarsal joint [see Subtalar, transtarsal or transmetatarsal joint]	Lower Extremity
70	Transtarsal joint [see Subtalar, transtarsal or transmetatarsal joint]	Lower Extremity
25	Transverse sinus	Head
26	Trigeminal nerve	Head
26	Trochlear nerve	Head
34	Tympanic membrane (ear drum)	Face
66	Ulna	Upper Extremity
64	Ulnar nerve [see Median, radial or ulnar nerve]	Upper Extremity
62	Upper extremity, whole area [use for Penetrating, Skin, Degloving, Amputation, Crush]	Upper Extremity
53	Ureter	Abdomen & Pelvic Contents
53	Urethra	Abdomen & Pelvic Contents
48	Urinary bladder [see Bladder]	Abdomen & Pelvic Contents
53	Uterus	Abdomen & Pelvic Contents
34	Uvea	Face
54	Vagina	Abdomen & Pelvic Contents
26	Vagus nerve	Head
	Vena Cava	
47	inferior	Abdomen & Pelvic Contents

Page	Anatomical Description	Section
41	superior	Thorax
	Vertebra	
56	cervical	Spine
61	lumbar	Spine
59	thoracic	Spine
25	Vertebral artery	Head
37	Vertebral artery	Neck
	Vessels	

Each body region, except the Spine and External, has a section titled Vessels. In addition to listing specific arteries and veins, a nonspecific description is included to code vessel injuries when precise information is lacking. The coder is urged to become acquainted with these default codes by body region.

Page	Anatomical Description	Section
34	Vestibular apparatus [see also Acoustic nerve in Head, page 26]	Face
26	Vestibular nerve [see Acoustic nerve]	Head
34	Vitreous	Face
38	Vocal cord	Neck
54	Vulva	Abdomen & Pelvic Contents
65	Wrist	Upper Extremity
35	Zygoma	Face

The following traumatic events to the whole body or to an entire body region are listed as follows:

Page		Section
74	Burns	External, Burns, Other
76	Electrical	External, Burns, Other
43	Hemothorax NFS [see Thoracic cavity NFS]	Thorax
76	Inhalation	External, Burns, Other
31-32	Loss of Consciousness (including concussion)	Head
43	Pneumothorax NFS [see Thoracic cavity NFS]	Thorax

●日本外傷学会 Trauma registry 検討委員会からのお願い

※本書の内容および翻訳に関する疑問等についてのご意見は，下記 URL にアクセスしてメールにて送信いただくか，へるす出版まで文書にてお寄せください。
また，本書発行後に修正すべき点が生じましたさいには，下記 URL にて告知いたしますのでご覧ください。
　へるす出版ホームページ URL：http://www.herusu-shuppan.co.jp/

| JCOPY | 〈(社)出版者著作権管理機構 委託出版物〉

本書の無断複写は著作権法上での例外を除き禁じられています。複写される場合は、そのつど事前に、下記の許諾を得てください。
(社)出版者著作権管理機構
TEL.03-3513-6969　FAX.03-3513-6979　e-mail：info@jcopy.or.jp

AIS90 Update 98 日本語対訳版

定　価
（本体価格10,000円＋税）

2003年10月16日　　第1版第1刷発行

監　　　訳　　日本外傷学会・財団法人 日本自動車研究所
翻　　　訳　　日本外傷学会 Trauma registry 検討委員会
発　行　者　　長谷川恒夫
発　行　所　　株式会社 へるす出版
〒164-0001　東京都中野区中野2-2-3
TEL　03(3384)8035（営業）　　03(3384)8155（編集）
振替・00180-7-175971

印刷所／広研印刷株式会社

落丁本，乱丁本はお取り替えいたします。　　　　　　　　　　　＜検印省略＞
©2003. Printed in Japan
ISBN　978-4-89269-455-4